Leber's Hereditary Optic Neuropathy

UNI-MED

UNI-MED Verlag AG
Bremen - London - Boston

Klopstock, Thomas:
Leber's Hereditary Optic Neuropathy/Thomas Klopstock.-
1st edition - Bremen: UNI-MED, 2024
(UNI-MED SCIENCE)
ISBN 978-3-8374-1673-2

Printed in Europe

MEDICINE - STATE OF THE ART

UNI-MED Verlag AG, one of the leading medical publishing companies in Germany, presents its highly successful series of scientific textbooks, covering all medical subjects. The authors are specialists in their fields and present the topics precisely, comprehensively, and with the facility of quick reference in mind. The books will be most useful for all doctors who wish to keep up to date with the latest developments in medicine.

The publisher would like to thank the company GenSight Biologics for supporting the production of this edition. The publisher assures that the industry partner could not influence the content of the book in any way, especially not therapy recommendations.

Preface

Leber's Hereditary Optic Neuropathy (LHON) is, in many regards, the prototype among the mitochondrial disorders. It was the first to be described in detail as a clinical entity, as early as in the mid 19th century. It was the first disease attributed to mutations of the mitochondrial DNA (mtDNA) in 1988, heralding the era of molecular mitochondrial medicine. It is the first (and still the only) mtDNA-associated disorder for which a therapy (idebenone) has been approved by the European Medicines Agency (2015). Gene therapy for LHON has also been the trailblazer among the mitochondrial disorders with several late-stage clinical trials already completed.

To date, we know quite a lot about the phenotype, epidemiology, natural history, genetic background, molecular pathomechanisms and treatment approaches for LHON. However, as it happens in science, the more we know, the more intriguing new questions arise, which need to be explored.

This book is meant to provide a comprehensive, albeit condensed, overview of our current knowledge as well as open questions and future avenues in LHON research. To this end, LHON experts from around the world gathered and worked together on the 11 chapters presented here. Of note, the international LHON researchers are a close-knit community of friends, which made the collaboration joyful and fruitful.

We hope that this book will convey the fascinating aspects of LHON and the research in this field to all readers, be they experts or novices. Moreover, we hope that ongoing pioneering LHON research will deliver more effective treatments for the LHON patient community.

Munich, July 2024 *Thomas Klopstock*

Authors

Piero Barboni, MD
Vita-Salute San Raffaele University Milan
IRCCS San Raffaele Scientific Institute
Milan, Italy
Chapter 5.

Valerio Carelli, MD, PhD
Department of Biomedical and Neuromotor Sciences (DIBINEM)
University of Bologna
Bologna, Italy
Chapters 1., 2., 3., 4., 9., 10.

Benson S. Chen, MD
John van Geest Centre for Brain Repair
E.D. Adrian Building, Forvie Site
Robinson Way
University of Cambridge
CB2 0PY Cambridge, United Kingdom
Chapter 11.

Rustum Karanjia, MD, PhD
University of Ottawa Eye Institute
The Ottawa Hospital
501 Smyth Road
Ottawa, Ontario, Canada
Chapter 6.

Thomas Klopstock, MD
Friedrich-Baur-Institute
Dept. of Neurology
LMU Klinikum, Ludwig-Maximilians-Universität München
Ziemssenstr. 1a
80336 Munich, Germany
Chapters 1., 10., 11.

Chiara La Morgia, MD, PhD
IRCCS Istituto delle Scienze Neurologiche di Bologna
Department of Biomedical and Neuromotor Sciences
University of Bologna
Via Altura, 3
40139 Bologna, Italy
Chapter 7.

Nancy J. Newman, MD
Department of Ophthalmology, Neurology and Neurological Surgery
Emory University School of Medicine
Atlanta, Georgia, USA

Chapter 6.

Berthold Pemp, MD, PD
Department of Ophthalmology and Optometry
Medical University of Vienna
Währinger Gürtel 18-20
1090 Vienna, Austria

Chapters 3., 10.

Claudia S. Priglinger, MD
Department of Ophthalmology
LMU Klinikum, Ludwig-Maximilians-Universität München
Mathildenstr. 8
80336 Munich, Germany

Chapters 5., 7.

Holger Prokisch, PhD
Institute of Human Genetics
Klinikum rechts der Isar der Technischen Universität München
Trogerstr. 32
81675 Munich, Germany

Chapter 8.

Alfredo A. Sadun, MD, PhD
Doheny Eye Institute and
Department of Ophthalmology
University of California, Los Angeles (UCLA)
Los Angeles, California, USA

Chapters 1., 2., 4.

José-Alain Sahel, MD
UPMC Vision Institute at Mercy Pavilion
1622 Locust Street, 15219
University of Pittsburgh School of Medicine
Pittsburgh, PA, USA

Chapters 11.

Sarah L. Stenton, MD, PhD
Division of Genetics and Genomics
Boston Children's Hospital
Harvard Medical School
300 Longwood Avenue, CLS 15023
Boston, MA 02115, USA

Chapter 8.

Catherine Vignal-Clermont, MD
Department of Neuro Ophthalmology Rothschild Foundation Hospital
Centre Hospitalier National d'Ophtalmologie des Quinze-Vingts
Paris, France

Chapter 6.

Patrick Yu-Wai-Man, MD, PhD
John van Geest Centre for Brain Repair
E.D. Adrian Building, Forvie Site
Robinson Way
University of Cambridge
CB2 0PY Cambridge, United Kingdom

Chapters 9., 11.

Contents

1. History of Leber's Hereditary Optic Neuropathy (LHON)

Thomas Klopstock, Valerio Carelli, Alfredo A. Sadun

1.1. First descriptions and definition of the disorder

German ophthalmologist Theodor Karl Gustav Leber (1840-1917) studied medicine in Heidelberg where he also did his doctorate in the group of physiologist Hermann von Helmholtz, the inventor of the ophthalmoscope. From 1867 to 1870, Leber worked as a resident physician in the Berlin eye hospital under the direction of Albrecht von Graefe, the founder of modern ophthalmology, and qualified as a professor in 1869. When von Graefe died, only 42 years old, from tuberculosis in 1870, Leber took over the temporary direction of the clinic. Soon after, he was appointed professor and director of the ophthalmology clinic in Göttingen (1871-1890), then held the same position until retirement in Heidelberg (1890-1910).

Theodor Leber is renowned for his meticulous descriptions of several ophthalmic diseases, and these were often first descriptions. In the case of Leber's Hereditary Optic Neuropathy (LHON), the sequence of reports is, however, somewhat ambiguous.

In fact, the first publication on a familial bilaterally blinding disease came from Albrecht von Graefe, later on Leber's teacher, in 1858 (1). He described three brothers who were all healthy until age 19 years, and then developed severe bilateral visual deterioration within weeks. The title of this publication, translated to English, is "*An unusual cause of hereditary amaurosis*", showing that von Graefe already recognized the genetic basis of this disease. The familial occurrence in males, the young adult age, as well as the dynamics and severity of the blinding process make it very likely that these brothers were indeed the first described LHON patients. Unusual, from today's perspective, is only the note that, according to von Graefe, all three brothers also suffered from headache at the onset of blinding symptoms.

Another report on a family with hereditary amaurosis was published in 1862 by English ophthalmologist W. Sedgwick as a very short communication (2). He described a family of 10 siblings where four of seven males but none of three females became blind between ages 42 and 56 years. Although this report is often cited as another early example of possible LHON, this must be doubted because the paternal uncle of the siblings was also affected by "amaurosis" which does not fit the LHON-like maternal inheritance.

The key publication, however, that eventually defined LHON is undoubtedly Leber's manuscript "*Ueber hereditäre und congenital-angelegte Sehnervenleiden*" (About hereditary and congenital diseases of the optic nerve) in 1871 (3). He described 18 patients from five families (including von Graefe's family above) and summarized the clinical characteristics as

- onset in adolescence or young adulthood (13-28 years), male predominance (16 of the 18 patients)
- acute or subacute onset of an often sequential but eventually bilateral visual loss
- rapid deterioration in the first 4 weeks, less rapid in the following months, then entering into a chronic stage
- severe loss of central visual acuity while the periphery is largely unaffected; Leber wrote about the five affected brothers in one family: "*Alle Brüder sind im Stande, sich auf der Strasse allein zu führen, können aber nicht mehr lesen.*" (corresponding to: All brothers can walk independently in the streets but cannot read any more)
- color vision affected
- in the chronic stage pale optic discs, starting on the temporal side
- optic nerve atrophy even if there is some clinical recovery (as in three of the 18 patients)
- brothers of unaffected mothers affected in two of the five families (an early hint to, at that time, unknown maternal inheritance)

Although Leber used the designation "*hereditary optic nerve disease*" in the title of his article and was obviously fully aware of the heritability of the disease, he also employed, in the body of the text, the terms "*retrobulbar neuritis*", "*neuroretinits optica*" and "*neuritis of optic nerve trunk*". By ophthalmoscopy, he noted some inflammatory signs which he considered, however, mild in relation to the severe visual loss.

1.2. Subsequent reports

In the subsequent years and decades, many cases and families were reported that may have represented LHON, as summarized in (4). The disorder was, however, assigned several different descriptive names (e.g., hereditary optic nerve disease, hereditary amblyopia, hereditary neuritis, familial retrobulbar neuritis), and it is not completely clear who first coined it as Leber's disease. A review by Kowalewski in 1906 on more than 70 families was titled "*familial optic atrophy*" (5), while another review by Nettleship in 1909 was titled "*On some hereditary diseases of the eye. Leber`s disease.*" (6). Of note, the latter author summarized hundreds of cases and reported a sex ratio of 300 males to 60 females. Wilbrand & Saenger in 1913 reinforced the typical signs of LHON, including onset in males around age 20 years, visual deterioration within weeks, and bilateral affection with an interval of up to 1.5 years between the eyes (7). Over the decades, numerous other studies characterized the clinical, epidemiological and laboratory features of the disorder, and only few can be mentioned here. Newman et al. in 1991 (8) and Riordan-Eva in 1995 (9) were two classics that helped define the disease landscape. Important characteristics of the disease included that men are much more likely to be affected than women. In America, Europe and Australia, 80-90% of affected were reported to be men (8, 10-12). An unusual aspect of this disease is the sudden sub-acute onset, typically about age 15-35 years with one eye following the other within a few months (8, 10-12). While the clinical course of LHON is dealt with in another chapter, it was usually described as deteriorating over a few months to about counting fingers vision. A central or central-caecal scotoma and severe dyschromatopsia were also characteristic for this disease. These features all pointed to the primary involvement of the papillo-macular bundle (PMB), something pointed out by Sadun and colleagues as highly suggestive that the pathological process targets the smallest fibers that constitute the PMB (13). Histopathology of LHON post-mortem tissues has born this out (14, 15). The prevalence of LHON was estimated to be around 1:45,000 in Europe (16).

1.3. Genetics

Due to the familial occurrence of the disorder, it was clear from the beginning and mentioned already by von Graefe and Leber in their initial reports that there was a genetic basis to the disease. Leber even noted in his seminal paper (3) that there were affected brothers of the unaffected mother of the index patients (all male) in two families, implying that the disease was inherited via the mother. Wilbrand & Saenger elaborated in 1913 (7) that the transmission occurs from healthy mothers to affected male children while they have healthy offspring. The fact that affected men have, without any exception, healthy children was already stressed by many early authors (17, 18).

While X-linked recessive transmission seemed to be the best explanation for the observed transmission pattern at the time, Meyer-Riemsloh already doubted in 1925 this hypothesis as he found the number of female carriers in an 8-generation pedigree too high for an X-linked disease (19). As early as 1936, Imai and Morikawi (20) surmised "*cytoplasmatic inheritance*" in Leber's disease through maternal oocytes, a revolutionary idea later reinforced by Ronne in 1944 (21) and Erickson in 1972 (22). Colenbrander in 1962 (23) and Wallace in 1970 (24, 25) speculated that this cytoplasmic agent could be a virus.

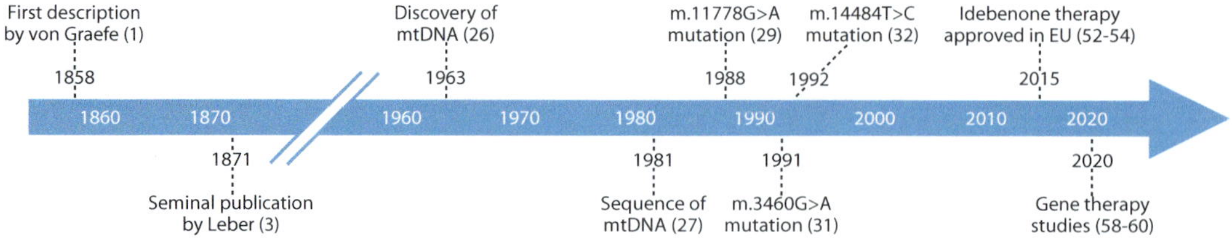

Figure 1.1: Timeline of major events in LHON research.

As so often happens, progress in basic science finally helped to understand clinical observations. The existence of mitochondrial DNA had been first reported by Nass & Nass in 1963 (26), and Anderson et al. published its complete sequence in 1981 (27). It is to the credit of Nikoskelainen and coauthors who drew the right conclusions and were the first to propose mitochondrial inheritance of LHON in 1984 (28). The breakthrough discovery was then achieved by Wallace and team in 1988, who identified a mutation at position 11778 of the mtDNA (m.11778G>A) as a cause for LHON (29). The year 1988 can be considered the starting point of molecular mitochondrial medicine due to the finding of this LHON mutation as well as to the discovery of mtDNA deletions as a cause of mitochondrial myopathy (30) as first reports on mtDNA defects leading to human disease. Thereafter, it was only a matter of a few years until the other two primary mtDNA mutations in LHON were identified: m.3460G>A in 1991 (31) and m.14484T>C in 1992 (32). Together, these three primary mutations account for >90% of LHON cases across the world. Their relative frequency differs somewhat between studies and countries but the m.11778G>A mutation is always the most frequent, e.g. 60/79 pedigrees (76%) in an English study (33), and 110/159 pedigrees (69%) in an international study (34). On average, the course of the disease is most severe in m.11778G>A and m.3460G>A mutation affected, and mildest in m.14484T>C mutation affected.

Rare mutations of the mtDNA, mostly also in complex I genes, may account for the remaining cases of LHON (35, 36) (www.mitomap.org). These can be identified by complete sequencing of the mtDNA which has replaced single mutation analysis as the primary diagnostic approach in many laboratories.

Sometimes, however, no mutation of the mtDNA is found at all despite a clear LHON phenotype. Many of these cases can now be explained by mutations in nuclear genes, transmitted in an autosomal recessive manner. Of note, the most relevant nuclear genes also code for complex I subunits (37), or for a newly discovered chaperone (DNAJC30) implicated in complex I turnover (38, 39).

1.4. Environment

The noxious effects of smoking on the optic nerve were already described in 1863 by Hutchinson (40) as "*tobacco amaurosis*", and even now so-called tobacco-alcohol amblyopia is in the differential diagnosis for LHON. Indeed, both tobacco and binge alcohol drinking increase the risk of clinical manifestation in LHON mutation carriers. The first mention of this association may be Hensen's publication in 1917 that described an increased LHON occurrence in soldiers of the World War I, and attributed it to exhaustion and heavy smoking on the battlefield ("*starkes Rauchen im Felde*") (41). From 1965, Wilson suggested that a defect in the conversion of cyanide to thiocyanate may cause the detrimental effects of smoking in LHON (42). This theory of a defective cyanide metabolism was later reinforced by several other groups (43-46). In 2001, an extraordinarily large pedigree of LHON with m.11778G>A mutation was found in a rural area of Brazil. Sadun et al. evaluated 530 eyes from 265 individuals of this 7-generation family, and found binge drinking of alcohol, and especially smoking to be important risk factors for conversion (47). In a seminal study, Kirkman et al. conducted a large multicenter epidemiological study of 196 affected and 206 unaffected carriers from 125 LHON pedigrees and found a strong and consistent association between visual loss and smoking, independent of gender and alcohol intake, leading to a clinical penetrance of 93% in men who smoked (48). In addition, there was a trend towards increased visual loss with alcohol, but only with heavy intake. Late-onset (after age 50 years) LHON patients had also significantly higher mean cumulative tobacco and alcohol consumption compared with unaffected carriers (49). Regarding the pathophysiological mechanisms, tobacco was found to trigger LHON by affecting mtDNA copy number, oxidative phosphorylation and ROS detoxification pathways (50). Based on these findings, asymptomatic carriers of a LHON mutation should be strongly advised not to smoke and to moderate their alcohol intake (48). Since vitamin B12 deficiency is also a known cause of mitochondrial optic neuropathy, it should be screened for in LHON mutation carriers and patients, and vitamin B12 supplemented when needed (51).

1.5. Treatment

Treatment approaches in LHON will be carefully dealt with in subsequent chapters of this book. However, some milestone studies should be highlighted here. Klopstock et al. conducted a prospective, double-blind, randomized, placebo-controlled trial referred to as the RHODOS clinical trial. This involved giving idebenone 900 mg/day or placebo (2:1 randomization) in 85 LHON patients for 6 months (52). While the primary endpoint did not reach statistical significance, secondary endpoints and post hoc analyses pointed consistently towards a clinical benefit of the drug. These results were bolstered by Carelli et al. in a retrospective analysis where LHON patients on idebenone treatment (n=44) had better outcomes than those without (n=59) (53). They also showed that the benefit of idebenone unfurled in many patients only after prolonged treatment suggesting that the RHODOS trial of 6 months was just too short (52, 53). A subsequent open-label, real-world study of long-term visual acuity and safety in 111 LHON patients treated with idebenone 900 mg/day showed, after an average treatment duration of 25.6 months, clinically relevant recovery in 46% of patients and clinically relevant stabilization (maintaining a visual acuity better than 1.0 logMAR) in 50% (54). This latter study indicated that prolonged idebenone treatment of at least 24 months is necessary before a patient is rated a non-responder, and again that the 6 months of the randomized trial (52) was too short to capture the full benefit of idebenone. Together, these studies led to conditional approval of idebenone for the treatment of LHON in the European Union in 2015, and it is still the only drug authorized for any mtDNA-associated disorder.

Retinal diseases such as LHON are ideal candidates for gene therapy due to the good accessibility via intravitreal or subretinal injections (allowing delivery of vectors in close apposition to the tissue of interest), and the presence of immune privilege (circumventing systemic immune responses). Accordingly, gene therapy for LHON due to the m.11778G>A mutation has been developed by several groups world-wide (55-57), all employing an adeno-associated virus type 2 vector carrying the wild-type ND4 gene, allotopic expression in the nucleus, and a mitochondrial targeting sequence to direct the ND4 protein into the mitochondria. Clinical trials showed bilateral visual improvement after only unilateral gene therapy injection which though desirable from patients' and clinicians' points of views was unexpected and precluded significance for the predefined primary endpoint, the difference between treated and sham-treated eyes (58-60). Further details are referred in the respective chapter of this book.

1.6. A glimpse into the future

Recent investigations are honing in on many aspects of LHON from genetics to epidemiology to clinical features to less clinically obvious psychophysical impairments in both affected and asymptomatic LHON carriers. There is growing excitement as new and powerful methodologies of science are applied to the problem of better understanding the molecular and atomic mechanisms. Progress is made in modelling the disease, from cell cultures to cybrids to mouse models to current approaches to building human retina organoids. Most importantly, there are several new and promising treatment modalities on the horizon beyond idebenone and gene therapy. The next decade promises to be very exciting with regard to basic and clinical research as well as therapeutic developments in LHON.

References

1. von Gräfe A. Ein ungewöhnlicher Fall von hereditärer Amaurose. Arch Ophthalmol. 1858;4:266-8.

2. Sedgwick S. Hereditary amaurosis. Medical Times and Gazette. 1862:309.

3. Leber T. Ueber hereditäre und congenital-angelegte Sehnervenleiden. Graefe's Archiv fur Ophthalmologie. 1871;17:249-91.

4. Schmidt D. Die hereditäre Leber'sche Optikusneuropathie (LHON). Düren: Shaker Verlag; 2020.

5. Kowalewski R. Familiäre Optikusatrophie. Zentralbl prakt Augenheilkd. 1906:114-5.

6. Nettleship E. On some hereditary diseases of the eye. Leber's disease. Trans Ophthalmol Soc UK. 1909;29:105-20.

7. Wilbrand H, Saenger, A. Die hereditäre Neuritis optica. Die Neurologie des Auges. 5. Wiesbaden: J.F. Bergmann; 1913. p. 135-72.

8. Newman NJ, Lott MT, Wallace DC. The clinical characteristics of pedigrees of Leber's hereditary optic neu-

ropathy with the 11778 mutation. American Journal of Ophthalmology. 1991;111(6):750-62.

9. Riordan-Eva P, Sanders MD, Govan GG, Sweeney MG, Da Costa J, Harding AE. The clinical features of Leber's hereditary optic neuropathy defined by the presence of a pathogenic mitochondrial DNA mutation. Brain. 1995;118(Pt 2):319-37.

10. Carroll WM, Mastaglia FL. Leber's optic neuropathy: a clinical and visual evoked potential study of affected and asymptomatic members of a six generation family. Brain. 1979;102(3):559-80.

11. Nikoskelainen EK, Savontaus ML, Wanne OP, Katila MJ, Nummelin KU. Leber's hereditary optic neuroretinopathy, a maternally inherited disease. A genealogic study in four pedigrees. Arch Ophthalmol. 1987;105(5): 665-71.

12. Mackey DA, Buttery RG. Leber hereditary optic neuropathy in Australia. Aust N Z J Ophthalmol. 1992;20(3): 177-84.

13. Sadun AA, Win PH, Ross-Cisneros FN, Walker SO, Carelli V. Leber's hereditary optic neuropathy differentially affects smaller axons in the optic nerve. Trans Am Ophthalmol Soc. 2000;98:223-32; discussion 32-5.

14. Pan BX, Ross-Cisneros FN, Carelli V, Rue KS, Salomao SR, Moraes-Filho MN, et al. Mathematically modeling the involvement of axons in Leber's hereditary optic neuropathy. Investigative Ophthalmology & Visual Science. 2012;53(12):7608-17.

15. Sadun AA, La Morgia C, Carelli V. Mitochondrial optic neuropathies: our travels from bench to bedside and back again. Clin Exp Ophthalmol. 2013;41(7):702-12.

16. Mascialino B, Leinonen M, Meier T. Meta-analysis of the prevalence of Leber hereditary optic neuropathy mtDNA mutations in Europe. Eur J Ophthalmol. 2012; 22(3):461-5.

17. Barth F. Ein weiterer Beitrag zur Vererbung der familiären Sehnervenatrophie (Lebersche Krankheit). Klin Monatsbl f Augenheilk. 1921;66:581-90.

18. Waardenburg PJ. Beitrag zur Vererbung der familiären Sehnervenatrophie (Leberschen Krankheit). Klin. Mbl. Augenheilk.73, 619 (1924). Klin Mbl Augenheilk. 1924;73:619-51.

19. Meyer-Riemsloh B. Über hereditäre Sehnervenatrophie (Leber). Klin Mbl Augenheilk. 1925;74:340-55.

20. Imai Y, Moriwaki, D. A probable case of cytoplasmic inheritance in man. A critique of Leber's disease. J Genetics. 1936;33:163-7.

21. Ronne H. The inheritance of Leber's disease. Acta Ophthal (Kobenhavn). 1944;22:203-13.

22. Erickson RP. Leber's optic atrophy, a possible example of maternal inheritance. Am J Hum Genet. 1972; 24(3):348-9.

23. Colenbrander MC. Observations on the heredity of Leber's disease. Ophthalmologica. 1962;144:446-50.

24. Wallace DC. A new manifestation of Leber's disease and a new explanation for the agency responsible for its unusual pattern of inheritance. Brain. 1970;93(1):121-32.

25. Wallace DC. Leber's optic atrophy: a possible example of vertical transmission of a slow virus in man. Australas Ann Med. 1970;19(3):259-62.

26. Nass MM, Nass S. Intramitochondrial fibers with DNA characteristics. I. Fixation and electron staining reactions. J Cell Biol. 1963;19(3):593-611.

27. Anderson S, Bankier AT, Barrell BG, de Bruijn MH, Coulson AR, Drouin J, et al. Sequence and organization of the human mitochondrial genome. Nature. 1981;290 (5806):457-65.

28. Nikoskelainen E, Hassinen IE, Paljarvi L, Lang H, Kalimo H. Leber's hereditary optic neuroretinopathy, a mitochondrial disease? Lancet (London, England). 1984; 2(8417-8418):1474.

29. Wallace DC, Singh G, Lott MT, Hodge JA, Schurr TG, Lezza AM, et al. Mitochondrial DNA mutation associated with Leber's hereditary optic neuropathy. Science. 1988;242(4884):1427-30.

30. Holt IJ, Harding AE, Morgan-Hughes JA. Deletions of muscle mitochondrial DNA in patients with mitochondrial myopathies. Nature. 1988;331(6158):717-9.

31. Howell N, Bindoff LA, McCullough DA, Kubacka I, Poulton J, Mackey D, et al. Leber hereditary optic neuropathy: identification of the same mitochondrial ND1 mutation in six pedigrees. Am J Hum Genet. 1991;49(5): 939-50.

32. Johns DR, Neufeld MJ, Park RD. An ND-6 mitochondrial DNA mutation associated with Leber hereditary optic neuropathy. Biochemical and biophysical research communications. 1992;187(3):1551-7.

33. Harding AE, Riordan-Eva P, Govan GG. Mitochondrial DNA diseases: genotype and phenotype in Leber's hereditary optic neuropathy. Muscle Nerve Suppl. 1995; 3:S82-4.

34. Mackey DA, Oostra RJ, Rosenberg T, Nikoskelainen E, Bronte-Stewart J, Poulton J, et al. Primary pathogenic mtDNA mutations in multigeneration pedigrees with Leber hereditary optic neuropathy. Am J Hum Genet. 1996;59(2):481-5.

35. Achilli A, Iommarini L, Olivieri A, Pala M, Hooshiar Kashani B, Reynier P, et al. Rare primary mitochondrial DNA mutations and probable synergistic variants in

Leber's hereditary optic neuropathy. PLoS One. 2012; 7(8):e42242.

36. Peverelli L, Catania A, Marchet S, Ciasca P, Cammarata G, Melzi L, et al. Leber's hereditary optic neuropathy: A report on novel mtDNA pathogenic variants. Front Neurol. 2021;12:657317.

37. Gerber S, Ding MG, Gerard X, Zwicker K, Zanlonghi X, Rio M, et al. Compound heterozygosity for severe and hypomorphic NDUFS2 mutations cause non-syndromic LHON-like optic neuropathy. Journal of Medical Genetics. 2017;54(5):346-56.

38. Stenton SL, Sheremet NL, Catarino CB, Andreeva NA, Assouline Z, Barboni P, et al. Impaired complex I repair causes recessive Leber's hereditary optic neuropathy. The Journal of clinical investigation. 2021;131(6).

39. Stenton SL, Tesarova M, Sheremet NL, Catarino CB, Carelli V, Ciara E, et al. DNAJC30 defect: a frequent cause of recessive Leber hereditary optic neuropathy and Leigh syndrome. Brain. 2022;145(5):1624-31.

40. Hutchinson J. Clinical data respecting amaurosis, more especially respecting that form of it supposed to be induced by tobacco. Lancet (London, England). 1863;2: 536-8.

41. Hensen. Über Neuritis optici hereditaria. Klin Mbl Augenhk. 1917;59:33-42.

42. Wilson J. Cyanide in human disease: a review of clinical and laboratory evidence. Fundam Appl Toxicol. 1983;3(5):397-9.

43. Cagianut B, Schnebli HP, Rhyner K, Furrer J. Decreased thiosulfate sulfur transferase (rhodanese) in Leber's hereditary optic atrophy. Klin Wochenschr. 1984;62(18):850-4.

44. Syme IG, Bronte-Stewart J, Foulds WS, McClure E, Logan R, Stansfield M. Clinical and biochemical findings in Leber's hereditary optic atrophy. Trans Ophthalmol Soc U K (1962). 1983;103(Pt 5):556-9.

45. Poole CJ, Kind PR. Deficiency of thiosulphate sulphurtransferase (rhodanese) in Leber's hereditary optic neuropathy. Br Med J (Clin Res Ed). 1986;292(6530): 1229-30.

46. Berninger TA, von Meyer L, Siess E, Schon O, Goebel FD. Leber's hereditary optic atrophy: further evidence for a defect of cyanide metabolism? Br J Ophthalmol. 1989;73(4):314-6.

47. Sadun AA, Carelli V, Salomao SR, Berezovsky A, Quiros PA, Sadun F, et al. Extensive investigation of a large Brazilian pedigree of 11778/haplogroup J Leber hereditary optic neuropathy. American journal of ophthalmology. 2003;136(2):231-8.

48. Kirkman MA, Yu-Wai-Man P, Korsten A, Leonhardt M, Dimitriadis K, De Coo IF, et al. Gene-environment interactions in Leber hereditary optic neuropathy. Brain. 2009;132(Pt 9):2317-26.

49. Dimitriadis K, Leonhardt M, Yu-Wai-Man P, Kirkman MA, Korsten A, De Coo IF, et al. Leber's hereditary optic neuropathy with late disease onset: clinical and molecular characteristics of 20 patients. Orphanet J Rare Dis. 2014;9:158.

50. Giordano L, Deceglie S, d'Adamo P, Valentino ML, La Morgia C, Fracasso F, et al. Cigarette toxicity triggers Leber's hereditary optic neuropathy by affecting mtDNA copy number, oxidative phosphorylation and ROS detoxification pathways. Cell Death Dis. 2015;6(12):e2021.

51. Zibold J, von Livonius B, Kolarova H, Rudolph G, Priglinger CS, Klopstock T, et al. Vitamin B12 in Leber hereditary optic neuropathy mutation carriers: a prospective cohort study. Orphanet J Rare Dis. 2022;17(1): 310.

52. Klopstock T, Yu-Wai-Man P, Dimitriadis K, Rouleau J, Heck S, Bailie M, et al. A randomized placebo-controlled trial of idebenone in Leber's hereditary optic neuropathy. Brain. 2011;134(Pt 9):2677-86.

53. Carelli V, La Morgia C, Valentino ML, Rizzo G, Carbonelli M, De Negri AM, et al. Idebenone treatment in Leber's hereditary optic neuropathy. Brain. 2011; 134(Pt 9):e188.

54. Catarino CB, von Livonius B, Priglinger C, Banik R, Matloob S, Tamhankar MA, et al. Real-World Clinical Experience With Idebenone in the Treatment of Leber Hereditary Optic Neuropathy. Journal of neuro-ophthalmology : the official journal of the North American Neuro-Ophthalmology Society. 2020;40(4):558-65.

55. Guy J, Qi X, Pallotti F, Schon EA, Manfredi G, Carelli V, et al. Rescue of a mitochondrial deficiency causing Leber Hereditary Optic Neuropathy. Annals of Neurology. 2002;52(5):534-42.

56. Pei H, Wan X, Hu W, Dong X, Li B. Construction and detection of a novel type of recombinant human rAAV2/2-ND4. Eye Sci. 2013;28(2):55-9.

57. Bonnet C, Augustin S, Ellouze S, Benit P, Bouaita A, Rustin P, et al. The optimized allotopic expression of ND1 or ND4 genes restores respiratory chain complex I activity in fibroblasts harboring mutations in these genes. Biochimica et biophysica acta. 2008;1783(10): 1707-17.

58. Yu-Wai-Man P, Newman NJ, Carelli V, Moster ML, Biousse V, Sadun AA, et al. Bilateral visual improvement with unilateral gene therapy injection for Leber hereditary optic neuropathy. Sci Transl Med. 2020;12(573).

59. Newman NJ, Yu-Wai-Man P, Carelli V, Moster ML, Biousse V, Vignal-Clermont C, et al. Efficacy and safety of intravitreal gene therapy for leber hereditary optic

neuropathy treated within 6 months of disease onset. Ophthalmology. 2021;128(5):649-60.

60. Newman NJ, Yu-Wai-Man P, Carelli V, Biousse V, Moster ML, Vignal-Clermont C, et al. Intravitreal gene therapy vs. natural history in patients with Leber hereditary optic neuropathy carrying the m.11778G>A ND4 mutation: Systematic review and indirect comparison. Front Neurol. 2021;12:662838.

2. Genetics of LHON

Alfredo A. Sadun, Valerio Carelli

2.1. Maternally inherited LHON and the role of mitochondrial DNA (mtDNA) pathogenic variants and haplotypes

Leber's hereditary optic neuropathy (LHON) is the paradigm of maternally inherited disorders (1, 2), which we now know are due to defective mitochondrial DNA (mtDNA) (3, 4). Maternal transmission of the disease has been described in the chapter on history of LHON. This was recognized early on as the hallmark of LHON inheritance in most families, though also characterized by incomplete penetrance and greater male prevalence (5, 6).

In 1988, the mtDNA analysis of LHON families was undertaken, as Sanger sequencing was available to completely decode the relatively small circular mtDNA molecule of about 16,5 kb (4) and compare it with the mtDNA reference sequence generated a few years before in 1981, the so-called "*Cambridge sequence*" (7).

In a landmark paper, Douglas Wallace and Eva Nikoskelainen reported the first mtDNA point mutation associated with LHON (8). This mutation, at position m.11778G>A/*MT-ND4*, remains the most frequent in populations of European descent (9-11) and it is even more frequently found in Asian populations with LHON (12-14). The second LHON pathogenic variant at position m.3460G>A/*MT-ND1* was reported simultaneously in Finland and in UK/Australian LHON families a few years later (15, 16). This showed genetic heterogeneity and also how pathogenic variants affecting different *ND* subunits genes of complex I may be similarly causative for LHON. That LHON was usually tied to complex I became further demonstrated with the identification of the third LHON pathogenic variant at position m.14484T>C/*MT-ND6*. This last variant remained initially overlooked as a possible cause in one LHON pedigree, despite it being recognized as a variant compared to the Cambridge reference sequence (17). The confounder in this family from Australia was the co-existence of other variants in the ND1 gene, which were also good candidates as being pathogenic, and in the setting of a very severe clinical phenotype. In fact, many patients from that family suffered infantile encephalopathy, some with features reminiscent of MELAS (18). Subsequently, the very same variant, m.14484T>C/*MT-ND6*, was recognized in LHON families characterized by the unusually benign feature of very high rate of spontaneous recovery of visual loss. This is now well-recognized as a hallmark for this mutation (19), as confirmed in multiple independent LHON pedigrees (20).

These three variants are now considered as the "primary" LHON mtDNA mutations, covering about 90 % of LHON patients worldwide (1, 2, 21). They are the necessary but not sufficient condition for developing optic neuropathy; then incomplete penetrance points to other factors being necessary for conversion of the disease to blindness (22). The primary LHON mutations occur as new mutational events on the mitochondrial genome and will segregate somatically in heteroplasmic fashion in human tissues; when heteroplasmy is below threshold levels, there is no clinical evidence of disease (4, 23). Furthermore, in the case of heteroplasmy, the germline segregation over a few generations will undergo a genetic bottleneck, which may lead to either their disappearance or the opposite, their establishment as homoplasmic variants (24-27). The large majority of LHON pedigrees are established homoplasmic maternal lineages carrying one of the three frequent LHON variants, thus heteroplasmy is not the explanation for incomplete penetrance in most LHON pedigrees (22). It must be noted that while both m.11778G>A/*MT-ND4* and m.14484T>C/*MT-ND6* LHON pathogenic variants are only rarely found as heteroplasmic, the m.3460G>A/*MT-ND1* variant has been frequently reported as heteroplasmic (Valerio Carelli, personal observation), raising the possibility of a different selective pressure against this specific variant. This last point needs to be firmly established by an appropriate survey of large LHON cohorts.

Over the years, with the transition from restriction fragment length polymorphism (RFLP) analysis to complete mtDNA sequencing that has become increasingly available and more systematically carried out for research purposes, the genetic variability of the mtDNA molecule beyond the specific "primary" LHON pathogenic variants has been taken into consideration in further investigations on LHON incomplete penetrance (1, 2). This line of investigation was favored by the expanding use of mtDNA genetic variability analysis for population and evolutionary studies (28, 29). A series of studies, with progressively larger cohorts of LHON probands analyzed, solidly established that while the m.3460G>A/*MT-ND1*variant is associated with LHON regardless of the mtDNA haplotype, both m.11778G>A/*MT-ND4* and m.14484T>C/*MT-ND6* LHON pathogenic variants are associated preferentially with the mtDNA J haplotype (30-34). Haplogroup J in populations of European descent represent approximatively 9 % of individuals (35), whereas in the largest study of 3,613 subjects from 159 LHON-affected pedigrees the m.11778G>A/*MT-ND4* LHON pathogenic variant was found in 28 % of cases associated with haplogroup J, and the m.14484T>C/*MT-ND6* in 99 % of the sample (34). This latter result for the m.14484T>C/*MT-ND6* variant is striking, and it is now understood that this variant may have very relevant founder events (36) and may have low (37) or essentially no penetrance when associated with non-J mtDNA backgrounds. In fact, it was recently estimated that in the general population the m.14484T>C/*MT-ND6* variant may be found in 1 out of every 800-1000 individuals without any relationship to LHON, thus essentially behaving as a population polymorphism (38, 39). Furthermore, evidence that the m.14484T>C/*MT-ND6* variant is the most benign was corroborated by the highest rate of spontaneous recovery of visual function occurring in these LHON patients (1, 2, 21).

The current interpretation is that the haplogroup J background constitutively carries a series of non-synonymous variants affecting the *ND* subunit genes (complex I), as well as a few others in the *cytb* gene (complex III), which may synergistically interact with the primary LHON variants to increase their pathogenic potential, possibly reflecting on greater penetrance. The role of the functional consequences of mtDNA haplotype J-associated polymorphic variants is still a matter of investigation: there is scattered evidence that this genetic background may in fact interfere with assembly and stability of complex I and possibly of supercomplexes (40), or interact with environmental factors, some of which relevant for LHON (41), as well as impinge on the general homeostatic control of mtDNA copy number (42). However, more work is needed before the mechanistic role of this specific mtDNA background is fully clarified.

In conclusion, given the moderate impact on complex I function of the three primary LHON variants (1, 2), their pathogenic potential may be substantially modulated by the mtDNA haplotype J, at least for m.11778G>A/*MT-ND4* and m.14484T>C/*MT-ND6* LHON variants, ultimately impacting on penetrance. It must be said that incomplete penetrance is not fully explained by the association with co-existing mtDNA variants, and the issues of exposure to environmental factors like tobacco smoking and the impact of nuclear DNA are likely to be important (1, 2, 21, 22).

Finally, about 10 % of LHON cases do not carry one of the 3 frequent LHON pathogenic variants: a long list of other variants, confirmed or of potential pathogenic role have been described in a few LHON cases and families (21, 43). The complex I *ND1* and *ND6* subunit genes are mutational hot spots for LHON (44, 45). Specific combinations of multiple polymorphic variants may also create a genetic risk for LHON, as firmly established by maternal inheritance of the phenotype and functional studies taking advantage of the cybrid cell model (46). There is also the infrequent occurrence of double troubles with two primary LHON variants coexisting (47, 48), as well as the presence of a primary LHON variant associated with other private or rare mtDNA variants of potential functional impact (49, 50). It remains controversial, as there is a dearth of functional studies, that would shed light on how double troubles differ in the clinical phenotype (51) or influence overall LHON penetrance (52, 53).

Practically, the main message for diagnostic purposes is that nowadays the complete mtDNA sequence analysis by next generation sequencing methods is the gold standard for understanding the mtDNA contribution to a maternally inherited LHON phenotype.

2.2. The new landscape of autosomal recessive LHON (arLHON)

Despite extensive mtDNA investigations, a small number of phenotypical LHON cases (less than 10 % in the European population) remains without any convincing mtDNA defect as revealed by complete sequencing (21). Moreover, many LHON cases are sporadic, or affected individuals may be restricted to the same generation, hence, not truly corroborating a maternal inheritance pattern. Thus, the report of a single family with a combination of heterozygous variants in a nuclear gene encoding for the *NDUFS2* subunit of complex I did not come as a complete surprise (54). Pathogenic variants in nuclear encoded subunits of complex I are a well-established cause of severe pediatric encephalopathies with the hallmarks of Leigh syndrome, but they also manifest with leukoencephalopathy or epileptic encephalopathy (55). Initially, this emblematic LHON case remained isolated until a large collection of patients with an LHON type of optic neuropathy was reported to carry a frequent recessive variant in the *DNAJC30* gene that encodes for a protein acting as a chaperone deputed to maintain complex I turnover (56-58).

A recent twist came with descriptions of arLHON cases due to variants in genes belonging to a pathway different from complex I, so far the key set of proteins responsible for mitochondrial dysfunction leading to LHON. In fact, pathogenic variants in the nuclear malonyl-CoA-acyl carrier protein transacylase (*MCAT*) gene were described first (59), followed by the report of a similar case with a homozygous variant in the mitochondrial trans-2-enoyl-CoA reductase (*MECR*) gene (60). Both *MCAT* and *MECR* genes belong to the same pathway for mitochondrial fatty acid synthesis (mtFAS), opening the new scenario of a possibly different pathogenic mechanism leading to an LHON-like phenocopy. However, the MECR cases were characterized by an unusual feature for LHON such as episodes of recurrent vision loss (60). Remarkably, allelic variants in both *MCAT* and *MECR* genes may also lead to the more severe Leigh syndrome or Leigh-like (DYTOABG [MIM: 617282]) clinical pictures (61-63), a feature that also applies to *DNAJC30* variants (56, 57) and rarely, to the primary LHON mtDNA variants (64, 65). For both *DNAJC30* and m.11778G>A/*MT-ND4* cases of Leigh syndrome, it was recently shown that the Leigh phenotype was the result of a digenic co-occurrence of heterozygous variants in nuclear encoded subunits of complex I, which may phenotypically modulate a shift to Leigh syndrome (57, 66).

In conclusion, arLHON has to be considered when mtDNA is excluded and whole exome sequencing should be undertaken to disclose the responsible gene. We predict that further cases will include novel genes belonging to complex I or mtFAS pathways; optic atrophy, with or without LHON features, is an emerging phenotype for these subgroups of genes (67).

2.3. Interacting genetic variants in both mtDNA and nuclear genomes: the digenic model

The epistatic interaction of mtDNA and nuclear genetic variants has not been well explored. The above-mentioned example of digenic inheritance for the variant phenotype of Leigh syndrome in association with mutations typically associated with LHON, seen with either the *DNAJC30* or m.11778G>A/*MT-ND4* genes, predicts that this scenario will occur again.

Chinese researchers have investigated how a digenic model may apply to the issue of incomplete penetrance in LHON. The first nuclear gene to be associated as a modifier of LHON incomplete penetrance was *YARS2* (68), followed by *PRICKLE3* (69). Variants in these two nuclear genes encoding for proteins essential to the efficient functioning of oxidative phosphorylation were found to co-segregate with LHON affected individuals in a few families from China carrying one of the primary LHON mutations. Functional studies corroborated the additional impact of these variants to the dysfunction driven by the primary LHON mtDNA mutation, thus supporting their role in this limited set of LHON families (70, 71). These examples suggest a digenic model similar to the previously mentioned case of Leigh syndrome that occurs with primary LHON mtDNA variants or *DNAJC30* gene mutations. However, so far the impact of both *YARS2* and *PRICKLE3* has not been reproduced in LHON families of Euro-

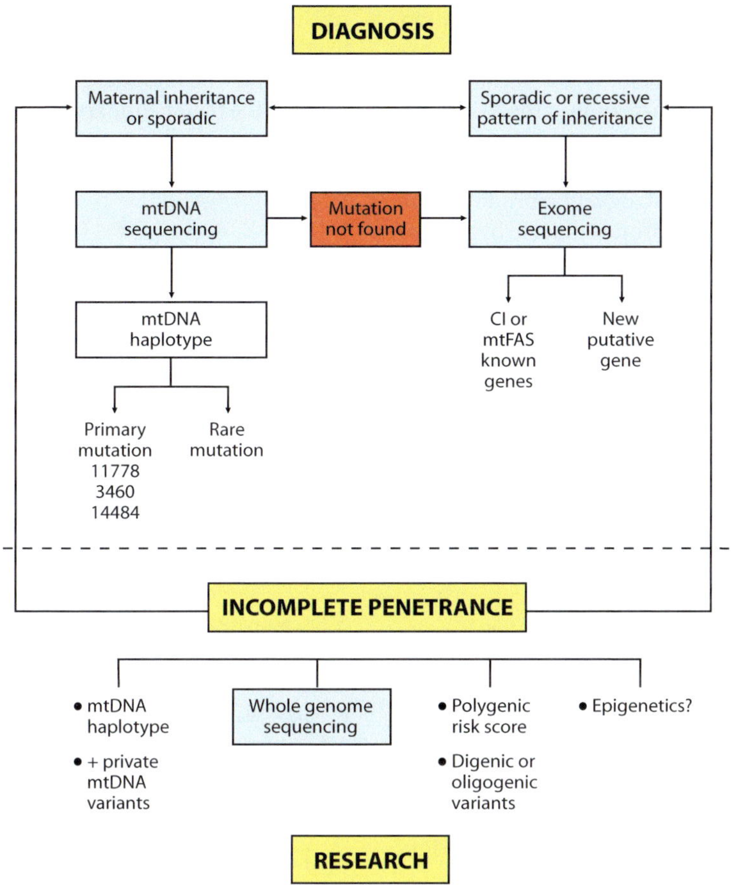

Figure 2.1: Schematic flow chart of LHON genetics.

pean ancestry. Thus, despite these reports, variable penetrance in LHON remains incompletely explained. The digenic model is an attractive one, but we cannot exclude even more complex scenarios. A burden of multiple variants in specific pathways may contribute to the development of optic atrophy and neurodegeneration. Such variants may be involved in complex I, mitochondrial metabolism or mitochondrial dynamics (72-74). They might also contribute to efficient compensatory mitochondrial biogenesis (75). Or they may all cooperate in the determination of the final degree of penetrance or even phenotype, implying the oligogenic contribution of multiple genes, as demonstrated for other diseases like ciliopathies (76). Parallel examples to LHON, characterized by homoplasmic primary mtDNA mutations, but with incomplete penetrance, are represented by the "*aminoglycoside-induced maternally inherited deafness*" associated with the mtDNA variant m.1555A>G/*MT-RNR1* (77, 78) or the so-called "*reversible Cytochrome-c-oxidase (COX)-deficiency*" associated with the mtDNA variant *m.14674T>C/MT-TE* (79, 80). In the first case, in the case of LHON, a digenic model has been proposed for a few families (81, 82), after accounting for aminoglycoside administration (79). For the latter disorder, variants in multiple genes along the same pathway related to mitochondrial translation seem to be the key contributory factor to disease penetrance, again in accordance with a digenic disease model (80).

2.4. Questions that remain to be conclusively resolved

Two major and interlinked questions need to be fully resolved in LHON genetics, which are male prevalence and incomplete penetrance (1, 2, 21).

Male prevalence has been considered for a long time as related to a hypothetical genetic factor on chromosome X, again assuming a digenic model (83, 84). However, neither study of the X-inactivation pattern in females carrying the primary LHON variants (85-87), nor gene linkage analysis (88-92) brought convincing and reproducible results supporting the chromosome X hypothesis. Only the *PRICKLE3* gene, previously mentioned as putative modifier in a few Chinese LHON families (69), is located on chromosome X, ultimately obeying the digenic model, but limited to a very small number of cases.

Interestingly, male prevalence seems to be associated with biochemical severity of the primary LHON mtDNA mutation, as the most penetrant in females seems to be the m.3460G>A/*MT-ND1* variant, and the less penetrant the m.14484T>C/*MT-ND6* (1); this suggests a functional effect better than a genetically determined trait (1, 2, 21). Following this line, the role of estrogens in ameliorating the LHON-related biochemical dysfunction has been documented in the cybrid cell model, mainly driven by the activation of mitochondrial biogenesis through the mitochondrial estrogen receptor beta (93, 94). This prompted the idea that a compensatory increase of mitochondrial mass may be beneficial in LHON, influencing penetrance in both genders (75). Ongoing studies are taking advantage of the technology that allows for reprogramming of somatic cells from LHON patients to pluripotent stem cells (iPSCs) (70, 71, 95) and further differentiation in retinal ganglion cells or retinal organoids and assembloids (96, 97). These investigations may lead to substantial advancements in understanding which genetic factors, besides the primary LHON mtDNA variants, may be most crucial in determining male prevalence, if any, and variable penetrance (98). In particular, the application of single cell analysis and multi-omic approaches will hopefully clarify the genetics of LHON, as well as the pathogenic mechanism.

Ultimately, the combination of these studies on the very cell type that is affected by the disease will be complemented by future studies of genome wide association and polygenic risk score approaches on large cohorts of LHON families. These will likely provide understanding and answers on how the nuclear genome variation may contribute to the risk for LHON, by examining gender preference, overall penetrance and cell-specific changes in phenotype. The ultimate goal will be to develop or advance the therapeutic approaches for LHON patients.

References

1. Carelli V, Ross-Cisneros FN, Sadun AA. Mitochondrial dysfunction as a cause of optic neuropathies. Prog Retin Eye Res. 2004 Jan;23(1):53-89.

2. Yu-Wai-Man P, Griffiths PG, Chinnery PF. Mitochondrial optic neuropathies - disease mechanisms and therapeutic strategies. Prog Retin Eye Res. 2011 Mar; 30(2):81-114.

3. Giles RE, Blanc H, Cann HM, Wallace DC. Maternal inheritance of human mitochondrial DNA. Proc Natl Acad Sci U S A. 1980 Nov;77(11):6715-9.

4. Schon EA, DiMauro S, Hirano M. Human mitochondrial DNA: roles of inherited and somatic mutations. Nat Rev Genet. 2012 Dec;13(12):878-90.

5. Erickson RP. Leber's optic atrophy, a possible example of maternal inheritance. Am J Hum Genet. 1972;24(3): 348-9.

6. Nikoskelainen EK, Savontaus ML, Wanne OP, Katila MJ, Nummelin KU. Leber's hereditary optic neuroretinopathy, a maternally inherited disease. A genealogic study in four pedigrees. Arch Ophthalmol. 1987;105(5): 665-71.

7. Anderson S, Bankier AT, Barrell BG, de Bruijn MH, Coulson AR, Drouin J, et al. Sequence and organization of the human mitochondrial genome. Nature. 1981; 290(5806):457-65.

8. Wallace DC, Singh G, Lott MT, Hodge JA, Schurr TG, Lezza AM, Elsas LJ 2nd, Nikoskelainen EK. Mitochondrial DNA mutation associated with Leber's hereditary optic neuropathy. Science. 1988 Dec 9;242(4884):1427-30.

9. Harding AE, Sweeney MG, Govan GG, Riordan-Eva P. Pedigree analysis in Leber hereditary optic neuropathy families with a pathogenic mtDNA mutation. Am J Hum Genet. 1995 Jul;57(1):77-86.

10. Rosenberg T, Nørby S, Schwartz M, Saillard J, Magalhães PJ, Leroy D, Kann EC, Duno M. Prevalence and Genetics of Leber Hereditary Optic Neuropathy in the Danish Population. Invest Ophthalmol Vis Sci. 2016 Mar;57(3):1370-5.

11. Fiorini C, Ormanbekova D, Palombo F, Carbonelli M, Amore G, Romagnoli M, d'Agati P, Valentino ML, Barboni P, Cascavilla ML, De Negri A, Sadun F, Carta A, Testa F, Petruzzella V, Guerriero S, Bianchi Marzoli S, Carelli V, La Morgia C, Caporali L. The Italian reappraisal on the most frequent genetic defects in hereditary

optic neuropathies and the global top 10. Brain. 2023 Mar 13:awad080.

12. Nakamura M, Ara F, Yamada M, Hotta Y, Hayakawa M, Fujiki K, Kanai A, Sakai J, Inoue M, Yamamoto M, et al. High frequency of mitochondrial ND4 gene mutation in Japanese pedigrees with Leber hereditary optic neuropathy. Jpn J Ophthalmol. 1992;36(1):56-61.

13. Yen MY, Wang AG, Chang WL, Hsu WM, Liu JH, Wei YH. Leber's hereditary optic neuropathy—the spectrum of mitochondrial DNA mutations in Chinese patients. Jpn J Ophthalmol. 2002 Jan-Feb;46(1):45-51.

14. Sathianvichitr K, Sigkaman B, Chirapapaisan N, Laowanapiban P, Padungkiatsagul T, Apinyawasisuk S, Witthayaweerasak J, Chuenkongkaew W. The epidemiology and mutation types of Leber's hereditary optic neuropathy in Thailand. Ann Med. 2022 Dec;54(1): 1601-1607.

15. Huoponen K, Vilkki J, Aula P, Nikoskelainen EK, Savontaus ML. A new mtDNA mutation associated with Leber hereditary optic neuroretinopathy. Am J Hum Genet. 1991 Jun;48(6):1147-53.

16. Howell N, Bindoff LA, McCullough DA, Kubacka I, Poulton J, Mackey D, Taylor L, Turnbull DM. Leber hereditary optic neuropathy: identification of the same mitochondrial ND1 mutation in six pedigrees. Am J Hum Genet. 1991 Nov;49(5):939-50.

17. Howell N, Kubacka I, Xu M, McCullough DA. Leber hereditary optic neuropathy: involvement of the mitochondrial ND1 gene and evidence for an intragenic suppressor mutation. Am J Hum Genet. 1991 May;48(5): 935-42.

18. Wallace DC. A new manifestation of Leber's disease and a new explanation for the agency responsible for its unusual pattern of inheritance. Brain. 1970;93(1):121-32.

19. Mackey D, Howell N. A variant of Leber hereditary optic neuropathy characterized by recovery of vision and by an unusual mitochondrial genetic etiology. Am J Hum Genet. 1992 Dec;51(6):1218-28.

20. Johns DR, Neufeld MJ, Park RD. An ND-6 mitochondrial DNA mutation associated with Leber hereditary optic neuropathy. Biochem Biophys Res Commun. 1992 Sep 30;187(3):1551-7.

21. Newman NJ, Yu-Wai-Man P, Biousse V, Carelli V. Understanding the molecular basis and pathogenesis of hereditary optic neuropathies: towards improved diagnosis and management. Lancet Neurol. 2023 Feb;22(2): 172-188.

22. Caporali L, Maresca A, Capristo M, Del Dotto V, Tagliavini F, Valentino ML, La Morgia C, Carelli V. Incomplete penetrance in mitochondrial optic neuropathies. Mitochondrion. 2017 Sep;36:130-137.

23. Howell N, Xu M, Halvorson S, Bodis-Wollner I, Sherman J. A heteroplasmic LHON family: tissue distribution and transmission of the 11778 mutation. Am J Hum Genet. 1994 Jul;55(1):203-6.

24. Barboni P, Mantovani V, Montagna P, Bragliani M, Cortelli P, Lugaresi E, Puddu P, Caramazza R. Mitochondrial DNA analysis in Leber's hereditary optic neuropathy. Ophthalmic Paediatr Genet. 1992 Dec;13(4): 219-26.

25. Harding AE, Sweeney MG, Govan GG, Riordan-Eva P. Pedigree analysis in Leber hereditary optic neuropathy families with a pathogenic mtDNA mutation. Am J Hum Genet. 1995 Jul;57(1):77-86.

26. Juvonen V, Nikoskelainen E, Lamminen T, Penttinen M, Aula P, Savontaus ML. Tissue distribution of the ND4/11778 mutation in heteroplasmic lineages with Leber hereditary optic neuropathy. Hum Mutat. 1997; 9(5):412-7.

27. Jacobi FK, Leo-Kottler B, Mittelviefhaus K, Zrenner E, Meyer J, Pusch CM, Wissinger B. Segregation patterns and heteroplasmy prevalence in Leber's hereditary optic neuropathy. Invest Ophthalmol Vis Sci. 2001 May;42(6): 1208-14.

28. Johnson MJ, Wallace DC, Ferris SD, Rattazzi MC, Cavalli-Sforza LL. Radiation of human mitochondria DNA types analyzed by restriction endonuclease cleavage patterns. J Mol Evol. 1983;19(3-4):255-71.

29. Cann RL, Stoneking M, Wilson AC. Mitochondrial DNA and human evolution. Nature. 1987 Jan 1-7; 325(6099):31-6.

30. Brown MD, Sun F, Wallace DC. Clustering of Caucasian Leber hereditary optic neuropathy patients containing the 11778 or 14484 mutations on an mtDNA lineage. Am J Hum Genet. 1997 Feb;60(2):381-7.

31. Torroni A, Petrozzi M, D'Urbano L, Sellitto D, Zeviani M, Carrara F, Carducci C, Leuzzi V, Carelli V, Barboni P, De Negri A, Scozzari R. Haplotype and phylogenetic analyses suggest that one European-specific mtDNA background plays a role in the expression of Leber hereditary optic neuropathy by increasing the penetrance of the primary mutations 11778 and 14484. Am J Hum Genet. 1997 May;60(5):1107-21.

32. Lamminen T, Huoponen K, Sistonen P, Juvonen V, Lahermo P, Aula P, Nikoskelainen E, Savontaus ML. mtDNA haplotype analysis in Finnish families with leber hereditary optic neuroretinopathy. Eur J Hum Genet. 1997 Sep-Oct;5(5):271-9.

33. Carelli V, Achilli A, Valentino ML, Rengo C, Semino O, Pala M, Olivieri A, Mattiazzi M, Pallotti F, Carrara F, Zeviani M, Leuzzi V, Carducci C, Valle G, Simionati B, Mendieta L, Salomao S, Belfort R Jr, Sadun AA, Torroni A. Haplogroup effects and recombination of mitochondrial DNA: novel clues from the analysis of Leber heredi-

tary optic neuropathy pedigrees. Am J Hum Genet. 2006 Apr;78(4):564-74.

34. Hudson G, Carelli V, Spruijt L, Gerards M, Mowbray C, Achilli A, Pyle A, Elson J, Howell N, La Morgia C, Valentino ML, Huoponen K, Savontaus ML, Nikoskelainen E, Sadun AA, Salomao SR, Belfort R Jr, Griffiths P, Yu-Wai-Man P, de Coo RF, Horvath R, Zeviani M, Smeets HJ, Torroni A, Chinnery PF. Clinical expression of Leber hereditary optic neuropathy is affected by the mitochondrial DNA-haplogroup background. Am J Hum Genet. 2007 Aug;81(2):228-33.

35. Pala M, Olivieri A, Achilli A, Accetturo M, Metspalu E, Reidla M, Tamm E, Karmin M, Reisberg T, HooshiarKashani B, Perego UA, Carossa V, Gandini F, Pereira JB, Soares P, Angerhofer N, Rychkov S, Al-Zahery N, Carelli V, Sanati MH, Houshmand M, Hatina J, Macaulay V, Pereira L, Woodward SR, Davies W, Gamble C, Baird D, Semino O, Villems R, Torroni A, Richards MB. Mitochondrial DNA signals of late glacial recolonization of Europe from near eastern refugia. Am J Hum Genet. 2012 May 4;90(5):915-24.

36. Howell N, Oostra RJ, Bolhuis PA, Spruijt L, Clarke LA, Mackey DA, Preston G, Herrnstadt C. Sequence analysis of the mitochondrial genomes from Dutch pedigrees with Leber hereditary optic neuropathy. Am J Hum Genet. 2003 Jun;72(6):1460-9.

37. Howell N, Herrnstadt C, Shults C, Mackey DA. Low penetrance of the 14484 LHON mutation when it arises in a non-haplogroup J mtDNA background. Am J Med Genet A. 2003 Jun 1;119A(2):147-51.

38. Watson EC, Davis RL, Ravishankar S, Copty J, Kummerfeld S, Sue CM. Low disease risk and penetrance in Leber hereditary optic neuropathy. Am J Hum Genet. 2023 Jan 5;110(1):166-169.

39. Mackey DA, Ong JS, MacGregor S, Whiteman DC, Craig JE, Lopez Sanchez MIG, Kearns LS, Staffieri SE, Clarke L, McGuinness MB, Meteoukki W, Samuel S, Ruddle JB, Chen C, Fraser CL, Harrison J, Howell N, Hewitt AW. Is the disease risk and penetrance in Leber hereditary optic neuropathy actually low? Am J Hum Genet. 2023 Jan 5;110(1):170-176.

40. Pello R, Martín MA, Carelli V, Nijtmans LG, Achilli A, Pala M, Torroni A, Gómez-Durán A, Ruiz-Pesini E, Martinuzzi A, Smeitink JA, Arenas J, Ugalde C. Mitochondrial DNA background modulates the assembly kinetics of OXPHOS complexes in a cellular model of mitochondrial disease. Hum Mol Genet. 2008 Dec 15; 17(24):4001-11.

41. Ghelli A, Porcelli AM, Zanna C, Vidoni S, Mattioli S, Barbieri A, Iommarini L, Pala M, Achilli A, Torroni A, Rugolo M, Carelli V. The background of mitochondrial DNA haplogroup J increases the sensitivity of Leber's hereditary optic neuropathy cells to 2,5-hexanedione toxicity. PLoS One. 2009 Nov 19;4(11):e7922.

42. Strobbe D, Caporali L, Iommarini L, Maresca A, Montopoli M, Martinuzzi A, Achilli A, Olivieri A, Torroni A, Carelli V, Ghelli A. Haplogroup J mitogenomes are the most sensitive to the pesticide rotenone: Relevance for human diseases. Neurobiol Dis. 2018 Jun; 114:129-139.

43. Achilli A, Iommarini L, Olivieri A, Pala M, Hooshiar Kashani B, Reynier P, La Morgia C, Valentino ML, Liguori R, Pizza F, Barboni P, Sadun F, De Negri AM, Zeviani M, Dollfus H, Moulignier A, Ducos G, Orssaud C, Bonneau D, Procaccio V, Leo-Kottler B, Fauser S, Wissinger B, Amati-Bonneau P, Torroni A, Carelli V. Rare primary mitochondrial DNA mutations and probable synergistic variants in Leber's hereditary optic neuropathy. PLoS One. 2012;7(8):e42242.

44. Chinnery PF, Brown DT, Andrews RM, Singh-Kler R, Riordan-Eva P, Lindley J, Applegarth DA, Turnbull DM, Howell N. The mitochondrial ND6 gene is a hot spot for mutations that cause Leber's hereditary optic neuropathy. Brain. 2001 Jan;124(Pt 1):209-18.

45. Valentino ML, Barboni P, Ghelli A, Bucchi L, Rengo C, Achilli A, Torroni A, Lugaresi A, Lodi R, Barbiroli B, Dotti M, Federico A, Baruzzi A, Carelli V. The ND1 gene of complex I is a mutational hot spot for Leber's hereditary optic neuropathy. Ann Neurol. 2004 Nov;56(5): 631-41.

46. Caporali L, Iommarini L, La Morgia C, Olivieri A, Achilli A, Maresca A, Valentino ML, Capristo M, Tagliavini F, Del Dotto V, Zanna C, Liguori R, Barboni P, Carbonelli M, Cocetta V, Montopoli M, Martinuzzi A, Cenacchi G, De Michele G, Testa F, Nesti A, Simonelli F, Porcelli AM, Torroni A, Carelli V. Peculiar combinations of individually non-pathogenic missense mitochondrial DNA variants cause low penetrance Leber's hereditary optic neuropathy. PLoS Genet. 2018 Feb 14; 14(2):e1007210.

47. Howell N, Miller NR, Mackey DA, Arnold A, Herrnstadt C, Williams IM, Kubacka I. Lightning strikes twice: Leber hereditary optic neuropathy families with two pathogenic mtDNA mutations. J Neuroophthalmol. 2002 Dec;22(4):262-9.

48. Catarino CB, Ahting U, Gusic M, Iuso A, Repp B, Peters K, Biskup S, von Livonius B, Prokisch H, Klopstock T. Characterization of a Leber's hereditary optic neuropathy (LHON) family harboring two primary LHON mutations m.11778G>A and m.14484T>C of the mitochondrial DNA. Mitochondrion. 2017 Sep;36:15-20.

49. Qu J, Li R, Zhou X, Tong Y, Yang L, Chen J, Zhao F, Lu C, Qian Y, Lu F, Guan MX. Cosegregation of the ND4 G11696A mutation with the LHON-associated ND4

G11778A mutation in a four generation Chinese family. Mitochondrion. 2007 Feb-Apr;7(1-2):140-6.

50. Wei QP, Zhou X, Yang L, Sun YH, Zhou J, Li G, Jiang R, Lu F, Qu J, Guan MX. The coexistence of mitochondrial ND6 T14484C and 12S rRNA A1555G mutations in a Chinese family with Leber's hereditary optic neuropathy and hearing loss. Biochem Biophys Res Commun. 2007 Jun 15;357(4):910-6.

51. Berardo A, Emmanuele V, Vargas W, Tanji K, Naini A, Hirano M. Leber hereditary optic neuropathy plus dystonia, and transverse myelitis due to double mutations in MT-ND4 and MT-ND6. J Neurol. 2020 Mar; 267(3):823-829.

52. Zhang S, Wang L, Hao Y, Wang P, Hao P, Yin K, Wang QK, Liu M. T14484C and T14502C in the mitochondrial ND6 gene are associated with Leber's hereditary optic neuropathy in a Chinese family. Mitochondrion. 2008 Jun;8(3):205-10.

53. Yang J, Zhu Y, Tong Y, Zhang Z, Chen L, Chen S, Cao Z, Liu C, Xu J, Ma X. The novel G10680A mutation is associated with complete penetrance of the LHON/ T14484C family. Mitochondrion. 2009 Jul;9(4):273-8.

54. Gerber S, Ding MG, Gérard X, Zwicker K, Zanlonghi X, Rio M, Serre V, Hanein S, Munnich A, Rotig A, Bianchi L, Amati-Bonneau P, Elpeleg O, Kaplan J, Brandt U, Rozet JM. Compound heterozygosity for severe and hypomorphic NDUFS2 mutations cause non-syndromic LHON-like optic neuropathy. J Med Genet. 2017 May;54(5):346-356.

55. Ferreira CR, Rahman S, Keller M, Zschocke J; ICIMD Advisory Group. An international classification of inherited metabolic disorders (ICIMD). J Inherit Metab Dis. 2021 Jan;44(1):164-177.

56. Stenton SL, Sheremet NL, Catarino CB, Andreeva NA, Assouline Z, Barboni P, Barel O, Berutti R, Bychkov I, Caporali L, Capristo M, Carbonelli M, Cascavilla ML, Charbel Issa P, Freisinger P, Gerber S, Ghezzi D, Graf E, Heidler J, Hempel M, Heon E, Itkis YS, Javasky E, Kaplan J, Kopajtich R, Kornblum C, Kovacs-Nagy R, Krylova TD, Kunz WS, La Morgia C, Lamperti C, Ludwig C, Malacarne PF, Maresca A, Mayr JA, Meisterknecht J, Nevinitsyna TA, Palombo F, Pode-Shakked B, Shmelkova MS, Strom TM, Tagliavini F, Tzadok M, van der Ven AT, Vignal-Clermont C, Wagner M, Zakharova EY, Zhorzholadze NV, Rozet JM, Carelli V, Tsygankova PG, Klopstock T, Wittig I, Prokisch H. Impaired complex I repair causes recessive Leber's hereditary optic neuropathy. J Clin Invest. 2021 Mar 15;131(6):e138267.

57. Stenton SL, Tesarova M, Sheremet NL, Catarino CB, Carelli V, Ciara E, Curry K, Engvall M, Fleming LR, Freisinger P, Iwanicka-Pronicka K, Jurkiewicz E, Klopstock T, Koenig MK, Kolárová H, Kousal B, Krylova T, La Morgia C, Nosková L, Piekutowska-Abramczuk D, Russo SN, Stránecký V, Tóthová I, Träisk F, Prokisch H. DNAJC30 defect: a frequent cause of recessive Leber hereditary optic neuropathy and Leigh syndrome. Brain. 2022 Jun 3;145(5):1624-1631.

58. Kieninger S, Xiao T, Weisschuh N, Kohl S, Rüther K, Kroisel PM, Brockmann T, Knappe S, Kellner U, Lagrèze W, Mazzola P, Haack TB, Wissinger B, Tonagel F. DNAJC30 disease-causing gene variants in a large Central European cohort of patients with suspected Leber's hereditary optic neuropathy and optic atrophy. J Med Genet. 2022 Oct;59(10):1027-1034.

59. Gerber S, Orssaud C, Kaplan J, Johansson C, Rozet JM. MCAT Mutations Cause Nuclear LHON-like Optic Neuropathy. Genes (Basel). 2021 Apr 2;12(4):521.

60. Fiorini C, Degiorgi A, Cascavilla ML, Tropeano CV, La Morgia C, Battista M, Ormanbekova D, Palombo F, Carbonelli M, Bandello F, Carelli V, Maresca A, Barboni P, Baruffini E, Caporali L. Recessive MECR pathogenic variants cause an LHON-like optic neuropathy. J Med Genet. 2023 Dec 21;61(1):93-101.

61. Achleitner MA, Hempel M, Tsiakas K, Feichtinger RG, Wortmann SB, Santer R, Mayr JA. Biallelic variants in MCAT in an infant with lactic acidosis, lipoylation disorder, and early death. In preparation.

62. Heimer G, Kerätär JM, Riley LG, Balasubramaniam S, Eyal E, Pietikäinen LP, Hiltunen JK, Marek-Yagel D, Hamada J, Gregory A, Rogers C, Hogarth P, Nance MA, Shalva N, Veber A, Tzadok M, Nissenkorn A, Tonduti D, Renaldo F; University of Washington Center for Mendelian Genomics; Kraoua I, Panteghini C, Valletta L, Garavaglia B, Cowley MJ, Gayevskiy V, Roscioli T, Silberstein JM, Hoffmann C, Raas-Rothschild A, Tiranti V, Anikster Y, Christodoulou J, Kastaniotis AJ, Ben-Zeev B, Hayflick SJ. MECR Mutations Cause Childhood-Onset Dystonia and Optic Atrophy, a Mitochondrial Fatty Acid Synthesis Disorder. Am J Hum Genet. 2016 Dec 1;99(6):1229-1244.

63. Gorukmez O, Gorukmez O, Havalı C. Novel MECR Mutation in Childhood-Onset Dystonia, Optic Atrophy, and Basal Ganglia Signal Abnormalities. Neuropediatrics. 2019 Oct;50(5):336-337.

64. Funalot B, Reynier P, Vighetto A, Ranoux D, Bonnefont JP, Godinot C, Malthièry Y, Mas JL. Leigh-like encephalopathy complicating Leber's hereditary optic neuropathy. Ann Neurol. 2002 Sep;52(3):374-7.

65. Fruhman G, Landsverk ML, Lotze TE, Hunter JV, Wangler MF, Adesina AM, Wong LJ, Scaglia F. Atypical presentation of Leigh syndrome associated with a Leber hereditary optic neuropathy primary mitochondrial DNA mutation. Mol Genet Metab. 2011 Jun;103(2):153-60.

66. Blickhäuser B, Stenton SL, Neuhofer CM, Floride E, Nesbitt V, Fratter C, Koch J, Kauffmann B, Catarino C,

Schlieben LD, Kopajtich R, Carelli V, Sadun AA, McFarland R, Fang F, La Morgia C, Paquay S, Nassogne MC, Ghezzi D, Lamperti C, Wortmann S, Poulton J, Klopstock T, Prokisch H. Digenic Leigh syndrome on the background of the m.11778G>A Leber hereditary optic neuropathy variant. Brain. 2024 Jun 3;147(6):1967-1974.

67. Lenaers G, Beaulieu C, Charif M, Gerber S, Kaplan J, Rozet JM. Autosomal recessive Leber hereditary optic neuropathy, a new neuro-ophthalmo-genetic paradigm. Brain. 2023 Aug 1;146(8):3156-3161.

68. Jiang P, Jin X, Peng Y, Wang M, Liu H, Liu X, Zhang Z, Ji Y, Zhang J, Liang M, Zhao F, Sun YH, Zhang M, Zhou X, Chen Y, Mo JQ, Huang T, Qu J, Guan MX. The exome sequencing identified the mutation in YARS2 encoding the mitochondrial tyrosyl-tRNA synthetase as a nuclear modifier for the phenotypic manifestation of Leber's hereditary optic neuropathy-associated mitochondrial DNA mutation. Hum Mol Genet. 2016 Feb 1;25(3):584-96.

69. Yu J, Liang X, Ji Y, Ai C, Liu J, Zhu L, Nie Z, Jin X, Wang C, Zhang J, Zhao F, Mei S, Zhao X, Zhou X, Zhang M, Wang M, Huang T, Jiang P, Guan MX. PRICKLE3 linked to ATPase biogenesis manifested Leber's hereditary optic neuropathy. J Clin Invest. 2020 Sep 1;130(9): 4935-4946.

70. Chen JR, Chen C, Chen J, Ji Y, Lian Y, Zhang J, Yu J, Li XY, Qu J, Guan MX. Nuclear modifier YARS2 allele correction restored retinal ganglion cells-specific deficiencies in Leber's hereditary optic neuropathy. Hum Mol Genet. 2023 Apr 20;32(9):1539-1551.

71. Nie Z, Wang C, Chen J, Ji Y, Zhang H, Zhao F, Zhou X, Guan MX. Abnormal morphology and function in retinal ganglion cells derived from patients-specific iPSCs generated from individuals with Leber's hereditary optic neuropathy. Hum Mol Genet. 2023 Jan 6; 32(2):231-243.

72. Petruzzella V, Tessa A, Torraco A, Fattori F, Dotti MT, Bruno C, Cardaioli E, Papa S, Federico A, Santorelli FM. The NDUFB11 gene is not a modifier in Leber hereditary optic neuropathy. Biochem Biophys Res Commun. 2007 Mar 30;355(1):181-7.

73. Hudson G, Yu-Wai-Man P, Zeviani M, Chinnery PF. Genetic variation in the methylenetetrahydrofolate reductase gene, MTHFR, does not alter the risk of visual failure in Leber's hereditary optic neuropathy. Mol Vis. 2009;15:870-5.

74. Hudson G, Yu-Wai-Man P, Griffiths PG, Caporali L, Salomao SS, Berezovsky A, Carelli V, Zeviani M, Chinnery PF. Variation in OPA1 does not explain the incomplete penetrance of Leber hereditary optic neuropathy. Mol Vis. 2010 Dec 15;16:2760-4.

75. Giordano C, Iommarini L, Giordano L, Maresca A, Pisano A, Valentino ML, Caporali L, Liguori R, Deceglie S, Roberti M, Fanelli F, Fracasso F, Ross-Cisneros FN, D'Adamo P, Hudson G, Pyle A, Yu-Wai-Man P, Chinnery PF, Zeviani M, Salomao SR, Berezovsky A, Belfort R Jr, Ventura DF, Moraes M, Moraes Filho M, Barboni P, Sadun F, De Negri A, Sadun AA, Tancredi A, Mancini M, d'Amati G, LoguercioPolosa P, Cantatore P, Carelli V. Efficient mitochondrial biogenesis drives incomplete penetrance in Leber's hereditary optic neuropathy. Brain. 2014 Feb;137(Pt 2):335-53.

76. Kousi M, Söylemez O, Ozanturk A, Mourtzi N, Akle S, Jungreis I, Muller J, Cassa CA, Brand H, Mokry JA, Wolf MY, Sadeghpour A, McFadden K, Lewis RA, Talkowski ME, Dollfus H, Kellis M, Davis EE, Sunyaev SR, Katsanis N. Evidence for secondary-variant genetic burden and non-random distribution across biological modules in a recessive ciliopathy. Nat Genet. 2020 Nov; 52(11):1145-1150.

77. Prezant TR, Agapian JV, Bohlman MC, Bu X, Oztas S, Qiu WQ, Arnos KS, Cortopassi GA, Jaber L, Rotter JI, et al. Mitochondrial ribosomal RNA mutation associated with both antibiotic-induced and non-syndromic deafness. Nat Genet. 1993 Jul;4(3):289-94.

78. Guan MX, Fischel-Ghodsian N, Attardi G. Nuclear background determines biochemical phenotype in the deafness-associated mitochondrial 12S rRNA mutation. Hum Mol Genet. 2001 Mar 15;10(6):573-80.

79. Horvath R, Kemp JP, Tuppen HA, Hudson G, Oldfors A, Marie SK, Moslemi AR, Servidei S, Holme E, Shanske S, Kollberg G, Jayakar P, Pyle A, Marks HM, Holinski-Feder E, Scavina M, Walter MC, Coku J, Günther-Scholz A, Smith PM, McFarland R, Chrzanowska-Lightowlers ZM, Lightowlers RN, Hirano M, Lochmüller H, Taylor RW, Chinnery PF, Tulinius M, DiMauro S. Molecular basis of infantile reversible cytochrome c oxidase deficiency myopathy. Brain. 2009 Nov;132(Pt 11):3165-74.

80. Hathazi D, Griffin H, Jennings MJ, Giunta M, Powell C, Pearce SF, Munro B, Wei W, Boczonadi V, Poulton J, Pyle A, Calabrese C, Gomez-Duran A, Schara U, Pitceathly RDS, Hanna MG, Joost K, Cotta A, Paim JF, Navarro MM, Duff J, Mattman A, Chapman K, Servidei S, Della Marina A, Uusimaa J, Roos A, Mootha V, Hirano M, Tulinius M, Giri M, Hoffmann EP, Lochmüller H, DiMauro S, Minczuk M, Chinnery PF, Müller JS, Horvath R. Metabolic shift underlies recovery in reversible infantile respiratory chain deficiency. EMBO J. 2020 Dec 1;39(23):e105364.

81. Li X, Li R, Lin X, Guan MX. Isolation and characterization of the putative nuclear modifier gene MTO1 involved in the pathogenesis of deafness-associated mitochondrial 12 S rRNA A1555G mutation. J Biol Chem. 2002 Jul 26;277(30):27256-64.

82. Guan MX, Yan Q, Li X, Bykhovskaya Y, Gallo-Teran J, Hajek P, Umeda N, Zhao H, Garrido G, Mengesha E, Suzuki T, del Castillo I, Peters JL, Li R, Qian Y, Wang X, Ballana E, Shohat M, Lu J, Estivill X, Watanabe K, Fischel-Ghodsian N. Mutation in TRMU related to transfer RNA modification modulates the phenotypic expression of the deafness-associated mitochondrial 12S ribosomal RNA mutations. Am J Hum Genet. 2006 Aug;79(2):291-302.

83. Bu XD, Rotter JI. X chromosome-linked and mitochondrial gene control of Leber hereditary optic neuropathy: evidence from segregation analysis for dependence on X chromosome inactivation. Proc Natl Acad Sci U S A. 1991 Sep 15;88(18):8198-202.

84. Bu X, Rotter JI. Leber hereditary optic neuropathy: estimation of number of embryonic precursor cells and disease threshold in heterozygous affected females at the X-linked locus. Clin Genet. 1992 Sep;42(3):143-8.

85. Oostra RJ, Kemp S, Bolhuis PA, Bleeker-Wagemakers EM. No evidence for 'skewed' inactivation of the X-chromosome as cause of Leber's hereditary optic neuropathy in female carriers. Hum Genet. 1996 Apr;97(4): 500-5.

86. Pegoraro E, Vettori A, Valentino ML, Molon A, Mostacciuolo ML, Howell N, Carelli V. X-inactivation pattern in multiple tissues from two Leber's hereditary optic neuropathy (LHON) patients. Am J Med Genet A. 2003 May 15;119A(1):37-40.

87. Hudson G, Carelli V, Horvath R, Zeviani M, Smeets HJ, Chinnery PF. X-Inactivation patterns in females harboring mtDNA mutations that cause Leber hereditary optic neuropathy. Mol Vis. 2007 Dec 21;13:2339-43.

88. Vilkki J, Ott J, Savontaus ML, Aula P, Nikoskelainen EK. Optic atrophy in Leber hereditary optic neuroretinopathy is probably determined by an X-chromosomal gene closely linked to DXS7. Am J Hum Genet. 1991 Mar;48(3):486-91.

89. Sweeney MG, Davis MB, Lashwood A, Brockington M, Toscano A, Harding AE. Evidence against an X-linked locus close to DXS7 determining visual loss susceptibility in British and Italian families with Leber hereditary optic neuropathy. Am J Hum Genet. 1992 Oct; 51(4):741-8.

90. Hudson G, Keers S, Yu-Wai-Man P, Griffiths P, Huoponen K, Savontaus ML, Nikoskelainen E, Zeviani M, Carrara F, Horvath R, Karcagi V, Spruijt L, de Coo IF, Smeets HJ, Chinnery PF. Identification of an X-chromosomal locus and haplotype modulating the phenotype of a mitochondrial DNA disorder. Am J Hum Genet. 2005 Dec;77(6):1086-91.

91. Shankar SP, Fingert JH, Carelli V, Valentino ML, King TM, Daiger SP, Salomao SR, Berezovsky A, Belfort R Jr, Braun TA, Sheffield VC, Sadun AA, Stone EM. Evidence for a novel x-linked modifier locus for leber hereditary optic neuropathy. Ophthalmic Genet. 2008 Mar; 29(1):17-24.

92. Ji Y, Jia X, Li S, Xiao X, Guo X, Zhang Q. Evaluation of the X-linked modifier loci for Leber hereditary optic neuropathy with the G11778A mutation in Chinese. Mol Vis. 2010 Mar 11;16:416-24.

93. Giordano C, Montopoli M, Perli E, Orlandi M, Fantin M, Ross-Cisneros FN, Caparrotta L, Martinuzzi A, Ragazzi E, Ghelli A, Sadun AA, d'Amati G, Carelli V. Oestrogens ameliorate mitochondrial dysfunction in Leber's hereditary optic neuropathy. Brain. 2011 Jan; 134(Pt 1):220-34.

94. Pisano A, Preziuso C, Iommarini L, Perli E, Grazioli P, Campese AF, Maresca A, Montopoli M, Masuelli L, Sadun AA, d'Amati G, Carelli V, Ghelli A, Giordano C. Targeting estrogen receptor β as preventive therapeutic strategy for Leber's hereditary optic neuropathy. Hum Mol Genet. 2015 Dec 15;24(24):6921-31.

95. Danese A, Patergnani S, Maresca A, Peron C, Raimondi A, Caporali L, Marchi S, La Morgia C, Del Dotto V, Zanna C, Iannielli A, Segnali A, Di Meo I, Cavaliere A, Lebiedzinska-Arciszewska M, Wieckowski MR, Martinuzzi A, Moraes-Filho MN, Salomao SR, Berezovsky A, Belfort R Jr, Buser C, Ross-Cisneros FN, Sadun AA, Tacchetti C, Broccoli V, Giorgi C, Tiranti V, Carelli V, Pinton P. Pathological mitophagy disrupts mitochondrial homeostasis in Leber's hereditary optic neuropathy. Cell Rep. 2022 Jul 19;40(3):111124.

96. Peron C, Maresca A, Cavaliere A, Iannielli A, Broccoli V, Carelli V, Di Meo I, Tiranti V. Exploiting hiPSCs in Leber's Hereditary Optic Neuropathy (LHON): Present Achievements and Future Perspectives. Front Neurol. 2021 Jun 8;12:648916.

97. Fligor CM, Lavekar SS, Harkin J, Shields PK, VanderWall KB, Huang KC, Gomes C, Meyer JS. Extension of retinofugal projections in an assembled model of human pluripotent stem cell-derived organoids. Stem Cell Reports. 2021 Sep 14;16(9):2228-2241.

98. Carelli V, La Morgia C, Ross-Cisneros FN, Sadun AA. Optic neuropathies: the tip of the neurodegeneration iceberg. Hum Mol Genet. 2017 Oct 1;26(R2):R139-R150.

3. Epidemiology

Berthold Pemp, Valerio Carelli

Leber's Hereditary Optic Neuropathy (LHON) is a rare disease, but among the inherited optic neuropathies it is one of the most common forms. Peculiar features of LHON are its subacute onset after a symptomless interval of variable length, a marked incomplete penetrance and a clear male bias.

3.1. Dependence on age and gender

LHON most commonly affects young men between the age of 15 and 35 years. However, all carriers of genetic variants predisposing them to LHON have a certain risk of becoming symptomatic any time from infancy to very old age, and irrespective of their gender. In a recent large demographic study collecting self-reported data from over 1.500 LHON patients worldwide, 25% of patients reported an age of onset below or above the typical age range, and about 25% of patients were female (1). Whereas males had a typical high peak of symptom onset between 14 and 26 years of age, the symptom onset in participating females was distributed more evenly across all ages with minor peaks in young adult and perimenopausal age (☞ Figure 3.1).

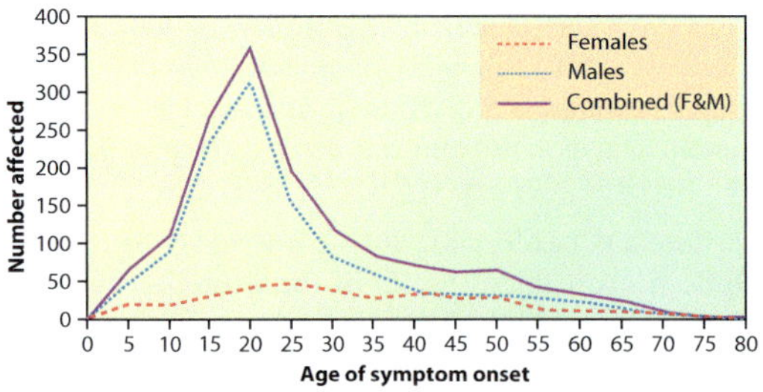

Figure 3.1: Age at LHON symptom onset (adapted from Poincenot et al. 2020 (1)).

Of course, the methodology of this study bears several limitations including possible accessibility, self-referral and recall biases. However, it enabled the aggregation of the largest dataset of LHON patients to date.

The evident higher susceptibility in young men results in an earlier mean onset age in male compared to female patients and in a general gender bias. Some studies in smaller cohorts showed up to 12 times more male patients (2-4). This could be driven by selection biases, population differences and the earlier misconception that LHON is a disease primarily affecting men, possibly resulting in less genetic testing in female patients with unexplained vision loss. Other national epidemiologic studies of LHON patients also show a male-to-female ratio of 3:1 (5, 6). So far, the cause of this gender difference is not proven, but may likely be related to hormonal differences, and possibly mediated by the stimulating effects of oestrogen on mitochondrial biogenesis. Interestingly, in patients younger than 5 and older than 45 years, there seems to be no clear gender bias (1). In addition, age distribution is similar when comparing patients with different pathogenic variants in the mitochondrial DNA (mtDNA).

3.2. Penetrance and prevalence

In pedigrees with LHON variants in the mtDNA, all members of the maternal lineage are at risk of developing the disease. However, penetrance can vary widely between families or even within different branches of the same family (☞ Figure 3.2).

Proportions of affected patients in different pedigrees ranges between 1% and 73% (6), and up to 65% of symptomatic patients have a negative family history of LHON (7). It has been observed that affected females are more likely to have affected children, particularly daughters, than unaffected female carriers (8). This indicates yet unknown additional pre-disposing factors in families with multiple cases. The overall lifetime risk for carriers of LHON variants to experience vision loss was previously estimated at 50% in males and 10% in females (8, 9). However, these numbers seem to be biased by families with high penetrance, in which LHON is more likely to be detected. More thorough pedigree analyses including multiple generations of familial and sporadic cases show a lower risk of vision loss. Of note, the majority of available LHON epidemiological data has been extrapolated from disease cohorts and is therefore subject to sampling bias. In a recent nationwide analysis of Australian pedigrees with identified LHON cases,

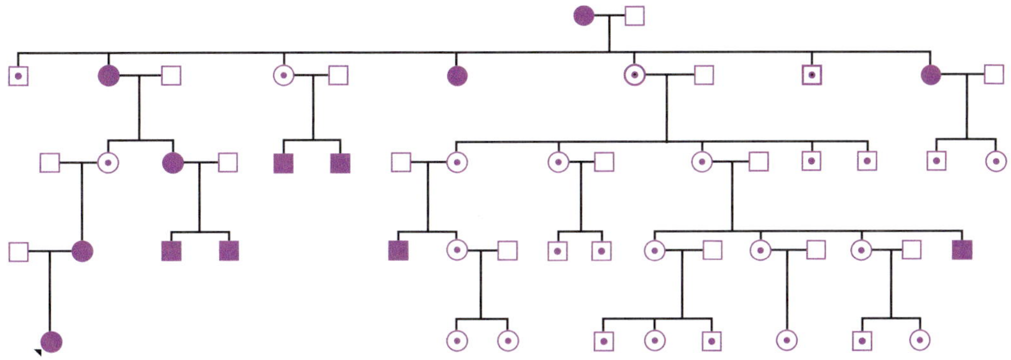

Figure 3.2: Pedigree scheme of a maternal line harboring the LHON variant m.3460G>A in the mtDNA. Filled symbols: symptomatic LHON patients; dotted symbols: asymptomatic carriers in the maternal lineage.

the overall penetrance in carriers of LHON variants was 17.5% for males and 5.4% for females (6). This indicated that on average only 1 in 6 males and 1 in 20 females in those families was at risk of developing vision loss. The calculated prevalence of LHON in this study was about 1 in 60.000 people. Other studies in confined geographical areas showed similar prevalence calculations from about 1:31.000 in the North East of England (5) to 1:50.000 in Japan (10), and 1:54.000 in Denmark (11). Combined data from the disease-based epidemiological studies in England, the Netherlands and Finland resulted in an estimated LHON prevalence of 1:45.000 in Europe (12). However, calculations based on disease cohorts do not represent primary epidemiologic data and may overestimate the true disease prevalence, since the frequency of individuals carrying a LHON variant in the general population is not reliably quantifiable from these data. Nevertheless, the prevalence of the presence of the three primary common LHON variants in the general population has also been estimated from disease cohorts by including unaffected family members of identified patients, and ranged from 1:4.600 to 1:15.000 (6, 13). The growing availability of large genetic databases now enables a better estimation of LHON variant carrier frequency in general population cohorts. This approach is less prone to a problematic selection bias and provides a more accurate understanding of disease risk and variant penetrance. In general population cohorts, LHON variants have been found considerably more often, in 1 of 350 to 1360 individuals (14, 15), resulting in an overall disease penetrance of 1-2% in carriers of LHON variants (16, 17), which is much lower than previously estimated.

Incidence data on LHON is even more sparse and only available from two survey studies in Japan, where the annual incidence was calculated as 1 new case per 1 to 2 million people (10, 18).

Interestingly, a decrease in penetrance and a decline in the risk of visual loss among pedigrees with familial LHON has been observed in large Australian and Brazilian pedigrees over the past century (6, 19). Since the genetic defect in the mtDNA was the same in all generations, other factors triggering disease conversion may have changed over time. The incomplete penetrance of LHON makes clear that the genetic predisposition is a necessary factor for the disease to occur, but additional genetic risk factors, hormonal factors as well as a variety of environmental triggers affecting mitochondrial function may play an important role. Tobacco smoking has been shown to be associated with a significantly increased risk of LHON, especially in patients above the typical onset age. A large retrospective analysis in 400 carriers of LHON variants showed an association between visual loss and smoking, with a penetrance rate of 93% in male smokers (20). Additional probable environmental triggers include excessive alcohol consumption, nutritional deficiencies, exposure to head trauma, organic solvents, pesticides or medications with known mitotoxic effects including antibiotic agents like linezolid and ethambutol or antiretrovirals (21). Unaffected LHON carriers should therefore be strongly advised not to smoke and to minimize their alcohol intake.

3.3. Genetic variation

Three different point mutations in the mtDNA account for over 90% of LHON cases. Most carriers inherit the predisposing variant from their mother, since de novo mutations are rare (5). Worldwide, the largest proportion (50-70%) of patients carry the m.11778G>A variant in the *MT-ND4* gene, followed by the m.14484T>C (10-30%) and the m.3460G>A (5-25%) variants in *MT-ND6* and *MT-ND1*, respectively (1, 22). Similar variant distributions are found in children compared to adult patients (1, 23). Interestingly, the m.14484T>C variant has been found more often in a large general UK population than m.11778G>A, implying a lower penetrance of LHON in the m.14484T>C variant (24). Conversely, m.3460G>A is rarely found in general populations, but has relatively high percentage in affected patients, implying a higher penetrance. Several other causative variants in the mtDNA are exceptionally rare (25). Similar to the three common variants, most of them affect genes encoding for subunits of complex I of the mitochondrial respiratory chain. However, some patients showing the clinical picture of LHON do not feature detectable pathogenic variants in the mtDNA. A comparably large number of such cases was recently identified to be caused by autosomal recessively inherited variants in the *DNAJC30* gene of the nuclear DNA, which encodes a chaperone protein necessary to maintain regular complex I function (26, 27) (☞ Chapter 8.).

Different proportions of causative variants can be seen in different world regions and ethnicities, most likely due to mutational founder effects. In the Far East the m.11778G>A variant is highly predominant with about 90% of all LHON cases (28, 29). In Canada, there is an unusually high prevalence (up to 86%) of patients with LHON carrying the m.14484T>C variant (3). The autosomal recessive form of LHON seems to be more frequent in Eastern Europe (26).

Some of the regional variability in penetrance could also be ascribed to differences in the mitochondrial genetic background on which the pathogenic mtDNA mutation is segregating. Combinations of specific benign mtDNA variants, known as haplogroups, which developed during human evolution, by themselves may influence the efficiency of the mitochondrial respiratory chain. In Caucasians carrying the m.11778G>A variant, haplogroup J seems to increase the risk of visual loss, whereas a lower risk was seen in the more common haplogroup H (21). Similarly, m.3460G>A carriers are more likely to experience visual loss if they belong to haplogroup K (25).

In a minority of pedigrees (15-37%), there is a copresence of mutant and wildtype variants, called heteroplasmy (5). Although the mutant load in optic nerve tissue cannot be assessed directly, a low heteroplasmy rate detected in other tissues could be a relevant factor, influencing the individual risk of penetrance in some family members. Some investigations suggested a lower risk of developing LHON when the mutation load in the blood lies below 60% (30). Other cohorts also showed a higher prevalence of the heteroplasmic state in unaffected carriers (14-37%) than in affected individuals (4-14%) (8, 31). However, the heteroplasmy rate in different tissues can vary considerably and affected patients can also present with low levels of LHON variants in blood cells. Hence, the risk of LHON in an asymptomatic individual with a heteroplasmic variant status cannot be directly determined. In addition, since heteroplasmy is not very common, it cannot fully explain the differences in disease penetrance between different LHON pedigrees.

3.4. Association with other diseases

LHON typically only affects the optic nerve, but additional features such as cardiac arrhythmia, peripheral neuropathy, and dystonia have been reported to occur more frequently in this disorder compared with the general population (25). Other, more severe deficits including spastic dystonia, ataxia, and encephalopathy can be found in a small number of so-called "LHON-plus" pedigrees, mostly with underlying rare variants in the mtDNA. Some patients also present with an overlap of LHON with clinical features of mitochondrial encephalomyopathy, lactic acidosis, and stroke-like episodes (MELAS) or Leigh-like encephalopathy. The co-occurrence of multiple sclerosis (MS) and LHON is also known as Harding's disease or LHON-MS (32). The patients show relapsing symptoms typical of MS including neurological symptoms, lymphocytic pleocytosis with oligoclonal bands in the cerebrospinal fluid and multiple white matter lesions in MR tomography of the brain. The loss of vision in LHON-MS often resembles symptoms of optic neuritis, it can be painful and episodical with temporary partial recovery, and often has untypically long intervals between the disease in both eyes. Like in MS, more women than men suffer from LHON-MS. Several studies suggested that LHON patients have a higher risk of developing MS (33, 34). The rate of MS in LHON patients is about 5% and therefore higher than in the general population. Genetically confirmed LHON in known MS patients was also found more frequently than expected (31). However, due to the rarity of both diseases, an increased incidence of LHON in MS cannot be precisely determined.

Conclusion

Some amount of information about the epidemiology of LHON has been obtained over the last few decades. However, the rarity of the disease, its great variability and the still incomplete knowledge of the exact pathophysiologic processes impede the research into important properties such as actual rates of penetrance and prevalence. Hopefully, future findings will also enable a more precise determination of the individual disease risk for carriers of LHON variants.

References

1. Poincenot L, Pearson AL, Karanjia R. Demographics of a large international population of patients affected by Leber's hereditary optic neuropathy. Ophthalmology. 2020;127(5):679-688.

2. Newman NJ, Lott MT, Wallace DC. The clinical characteristics of pedigrees of Leber's hereditary optic neuropathy with the 11778 mutation. Am J Ophthalmol. 1991;111(6):750-762.

3. Macmillan C, Kirkham T, Fu K, Allison V, Andermann E, Chitayat D, Fortier D, Gans M, Hare H, Quercia N, Zackon D, Shoubridge EA. Pedigree analysis of French Canadian families with T14484C Leber's hereditary optic neuropathy. Neurology. 1998;50(2):417-422.

4. Maciel-Guerra AT, Zanchetta LM, Amaral Fernandes MS, Andrade PB, do Amor Divino Miranda PM, Sartorato EL. Leber's hereditary optic neuropathy: clinical and molecular profile of a Brazilian sample. Ophthalmic Genet. 2010;31(3):126-128.

5. Yu-Wai-Man P, Griffiths PG, Brown DT, Howell N, Turnbull DM, Chinnery PF. The epidemiology of Leber hereditary optic neuropathy in the North East of England. Am J Hum Genet. 2003;72(2):333-339.

6. Lopez Sanchez MIG, Kearns LS, Staffieri SE, Clarke L, McGuinness MB, Meteoukki W, Samuel S, Ruddle JB, Chen C, Fraser CL, Harrison J, Hewitt AW, Howell N, Mackey DA. Establishing risk of vision loss in Leber hereditary optic neuropathy. Am J Hum Genet. 2021;108 (11):2159-2170.

7. Jia X, Li S, Xiao X, Guo X, Zhang Q. Molecular epidemiology of mtDNA mutations in 903 Chinese families suspected with Leber hereditary optic neuropathy. J Hum Genet. 2006;51(10):851-856.

8. Harding AE, Sweeney MG, Govan GG, Riordan-Eva P. Pedigree analysis in Leber hereditary optic neuropathy families with a pathogenic mtDNA mutation. Am J Hum Genet. 1995;57(1):77-86.

9. Riordan-Eva P, Sanders MD, Govan GG, Sweeney MG, Da Costa J, Harding AE. The clinical features of Leber's hereditary optic neuropathy defined by the presence of a pathogenic mitochondrial DNA mutation. Brain. 1995;118 (2):319-337.

10. Takano F, Ueda K, Godefrooij DA, Yamagami A, Ishikawa H, Chuman H, Ishikawa H, Ikeda Y, Sakamoto T, Nakamura M. Incidence of Leber hereditary optic neuropathy in 2019 in Japan: a second nationwide questionnaire survey. Orphanet J Rare Dis. 2022;17(1):319.

11. Rosenberg T, Nørby S, Schwartz M, Saillard J, Magalhães PJ, Leroy D, Kann EC, Duno M. Prevalence and genetics of Leber hereditary optic neuropathy in the danish population. Invest Ophthalmol Vis Sci. 2016;57(3): 1370-1375.

12. Mascialino B, Leinonen M, Meier T. Meta-analysis of the prevalence of Leber hereditary optic neuropathy mtDNA mutations in Europe. Eur J Ophthalmol. 2012; 22(3):461-465.

13. Chinnery PF, Johnson MA, Wardell TM, Singh-Kler R, Hayes C, Brown DT, Taylor RW, Bindoff LA, Turnbull DM. The epidemiology of pathogenic mitochondrial DNA mutations. Ann Neurol. 2000;48(2):188-193.

14. Elliott HR, Samuels DC, Eden JA, Relton CL, Chinnery PF. Pathogenic mitochondrial DNA mutations are common in the general population. Am J Hum Genet. 2008;83(2):254-260.

15. Laricchia KM, Lake NJ, Watts NA, Shand M, Haessly A, Gauthier L, Benjamin D, Banks E, Soto J, Garimella K, Emery J; Genome Aggregation Database Consortium; Rehm HL, MacArthur DG, Tiao G, Lek M, Mootha VK, Calvo SE. Mitochondrial DNA variation across 56,434 individuals in gnomAD. Genome Res. 2022;32(3):569-582.

16. Watson EC, Davis RL, Ravishankar S, Copty J, Kummerfeld S, Sue CM. Low disease risk and penetrance in Leber hereditary optic neuropathy. Am J Hum Genet. 2023;110(1):166-169.

17. Mackey DA, Ong JS, MacGregor S, Whiteman DC, Craig JE, Lopez Sanchez MIG, Kearns LS, Staffieri SE, Clarke L, McGuinness MB, Meteoukki W, Samuel S, Ruddle JB, Chen C, Fraser CL, Harrison J, Howell N, Hewitt AW. Is the disease risk and penetrance in Leber hereditary optic neuropathy actually low? Am J Hum Genet. 2023;110(1):170-176.

18. Ueda K, Morizane Y, Shiraga F, Shikishima K, Ishikawa H, Wakakura M, Nakamura M. Nationwide epidemiological survey of Leber hereditary optic neuropathy in Japan. J Epidemiol. 2017;27(9):447-450.

19. Sadun AA, Carelli V, Salomao SR, Berezovsky A, Quiros PA, Sadun F, DeNegri AM, Andrade R, Moraes M, Passos A, Kjaer P, Pereira J, Valentino ML, Schein S, Belfort R. Extensive investigation of a large Brazilian pedigree of 11778/haplogroup J Leber hereditary optic neuropathy. Am J Ophthalmol. 2003;136(2):231-238.

20. Kirkman MA, Yu-Wai-Man P, Korsten A, Leonhardt M, Dimitriadis K, De Coo IF, Klopstock T, Chinnery PF. Gene-environment interactions in Leber hereditary optic neuropathy. Brain. 2009;132(Pt 9):2317-2326.

21. Caporali L, Maresca A, Capristo M, Del Dotto V, Tagliavini F, Valentino ML, La Morgia C, Carelli V. Incomplete penetrance in mitochondrial optic neuropathies. Mitochondrion. 2017;36:130-137.

22. Newman NJ. Leber's hereditary optic neuropathy. New genetic considerations. Arch Neurol. 1993;50(5): 540-548.

23. Majander A, Bowman R, Poulton J, Antcliff RJ, Reddy MA, Michaelides M, Webster AR, Chinnery PF, Votruba M, Moore AT, Yu-Wai-Man P. Childhood-onset Leber hereditary optic neuropathy. Br J Ophthalmol. 2017;101(11):1505-1509.

24. Yonova-Doing E, Calabrese C, Gomez-Duran A, Schon K, Wei W, Karthikeyan S, Chinnery PF, Howson JMM. An atlas of mitochondrial DNA genotype-phenotype associations in the UK Biobank. Nat Genet. 2021; 53(7):982-993.

25. Yu-Wai-Man P, Griffiths PG, Chinnery PF. Mitochondrial optic neuropathies - disease mechanisms and therapeutic strategies. Prog Retin Eye Res. 2011;30(2): 81-114.

26. Stenton SL, Sheremet NL, Catarino CB, Andreeva NA, Assouline Z, Barboni P, Barel O, Berutti R, Bychkov I, Caporali L, Capristo M, Carbonelli M, Cascavilla ML, Charbel Issa P, Freisinger P, Gerber S, Ghezzi D, Graf E, Heidler J, Hempel M, Heon E, Itkis YS, Javasky E, Kaplan J, Kopajtich R, Kornblum C, Kovacs-Nagy R, Krylova TD, Kunz WS, La Morgia C, Lamperti C, Ludwig C, Malacarne PF, Maresca A, Mayr JA, Meisterknecht J, Nevinitsyna TA, Palombo F, Pode-Shakked B, Shmelkova MS, Strom TM, Tagliavini F, Tzadok M, van der Ven AT, Vignal-Clermont C, Wagner M, Zakharova EY, Zhorzholadze NV, Rozet JM, Carelli V, Tsygankova PG, Klopstock T, Wittig I, Prokisch H. Impaired complex I repair causes recessive Leber's hereditary optic neuropathy. J Clin Invest. 2021;131(6):e138267.

27. Skorczyk-Werner A, Tonska K, Maciejczuk A, Nowomiejska K, Korwin M, Oldak M, Wawrocka A, Krawczynski MR. DNAJC30 Gene Variants Are a Frequent Cause of a Rare Disease: Leber Hereditary Optic Neuropathy in Polish Patients. Int J Mol Sci. 2023;24(24):17496.

28. Mashima Y, Yamada K, Wakakura M, Kigasawa K, Kudoh J, Shimizu N, Oguchi Y. Spectrum of pathogenic mitochondrial DNA mutations and clinical features in Japanese families with Leber's hereditary optic neuropathy. Curr Eye Res. 1998;17(4):403-408.

29. Sathianvichitr K, Sigkaman B, Chirapapaisan N, Laowanapiban P, Padungkiatsagul T, Apinyawasisuk S, Witthayaweerasak J, Chuenkongkaew W. The epidemiology and mutation types of Leber's hereditary optic neuropathy in Thailand. Ann Med. 2022;54(1):1601-1607.

30. Chinnery PF, Andrews RM, Turnbull DM, Howell NN. Leber hereditary optic neuropathy: Does heteroplasmy influence the inheritance and expression of the G11778A mitochondrial DNA mutation? Am J Med Genet. 2001;98(3):235-243.

31. Phasukkijwatana N, Chuenkongkaew WL, Suphavilai R, Suktitipat B, Pingsuthiwong S, Ruangvaravate N, Atchaneeyasakul LO, Warrasak S, Poonyathalang A, Sura T, Lertrit P. The unique characteristics of Thai Leber hereditary optic neuropathy: analysis of 30 G11778A pedigrees. J Hum Genet. 2006;51(4):298-304.

32. Pfeffer G, Burke A, Yu-Wai-Man P, Compston DA, Chinnery PF. Clinical features of MS associated with Leber hereditary optic neuropathy mtDNA mutations. Neurology. 2013;81(24):2073-2081.

33. Vanopdenbosch L, Dubois B, D'Hooghe MB, Meire F, Carton H. Mitochondrial mutations of Leber's hereditary optic neuropathy: a risk factor for multiple sclerosis. J Neurol. 2000;247(7):535-543.

34. Vestergaard N, Rosenberg T, Torp-Pedersen C, Vorum H, Andersen CU, Aasbjerg K. Increased mortality and comorbidity associated with Leber's hereditary optic neuropathy: A nationwide cohort study. Invest Ophthalmol Vis Sci. 2017;58(11):4586-4592.

4. Molecular background and pathophysiology of LHON

Alfredo A. Sadun, Valerio Carelli

4.1. From mtDNA mutations to complex I dysfunction

The three most common mitochondrial DNA (mtDNA) mutations associated with Leber's hereditary optic neuropathy (LHON), as well as the large majority of the rarer mtDNA mutations and most of the nuclear DNA recessive mutations, almost invariably affect complex I (1). We here mostly focus on the three common mtDNA variants affecting the ND1 gene (*m.3460G>A*), ND4 gene (*m.11778G>A*), and ND6 gene (*m.14484T>C*), all encoding for complex I subunits.

Complex I is the entry point of the electron flow feeding the mitochondrial electron transport chain which, through a series of redox reactions, allows for mitochondrial respiration, energy conservations and ultimately ATP synthesis through oxidative phosphorylation (☞ Figure 4.1). Complex I, as well as complexes III, IV and V are all composed of many protein subunits, the large majority coded by nuclear DNA, and only 13 being encoded by mtDNA. Complex I consists of 45 subunits, 7 of which are mtDNA encoded (2), and a growing number of ancillary factors involved in assembly and turnover of this very large enzyme (3). Complex I (a NADH:Ubiquinone oxidoreductase) couples the energy released from the electron transfer needed to reduce coenzyme Q 10 (ubiquinone; CoQ) with proton translocation across the mitochondrial inner membrane (4). Now that the cryo-EM structure of complex I provided key information to understand its function (5), it became clearer that out of the 3 common mtDNA variants associated with LHON only the *m.3460G>A* change significantly reduces complex I redox activity by affecting the ND1 subunit,

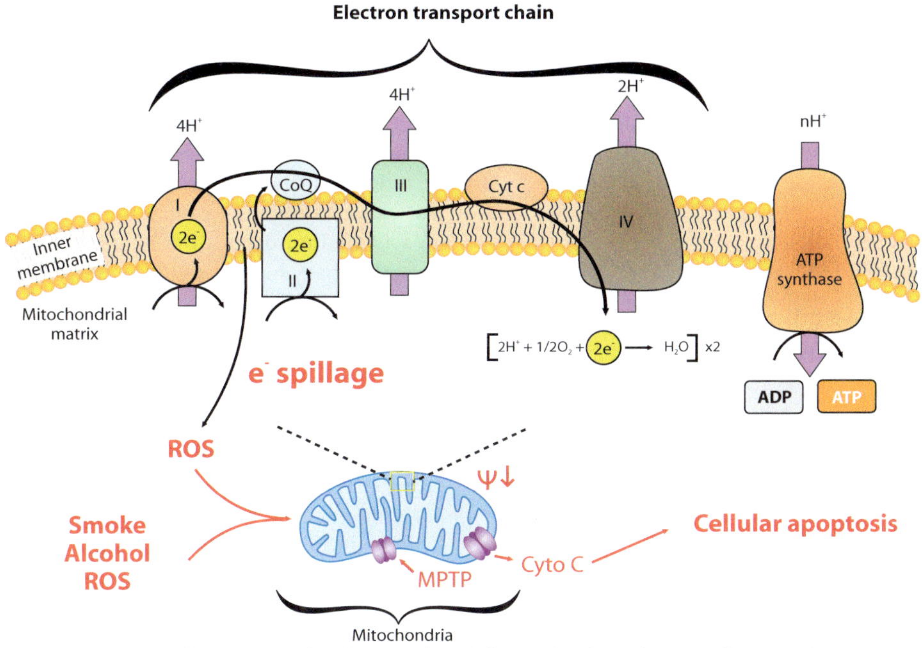

Figure 4.1: Electron transfer occurs in this diagram from left to right along the complexes, and energy is stored as a proton gradient that drives ATP production. LHON mutations produce a minor decrease of ATP production but also a much greater production of ROS (ref. [2]). ROS lower the electrical potential across the mitochondrial membrane which, in turn, leads to opening of the mitochondrial permeability transition pore (MPTP) initiating apoptosis of the RGC (ref. [4]). Adapted from ref. (3).

which participates to the CoQ binding pocket (4, 5). The other two LHON mtDNA pathogenic variants, *m.11778G>A* and *m.14484T>C*, by affecting respectively the ND4 and ND6 subunits, most probably affect the proton translocation activity and only slightly affect complex I redox activity (4-7). However, if instead of using the spectrophotometric assessment of electron flow and CoQ reduction (6, 7), we measure the ATP synthesis driven by complex I substrates or if we measure oxygen consumption, all three mutations clearly impair complex I function, reducing the bioenergetic efficiency (8, 9), increasing the production of reactive oxygen species (ROS) (10, 11) and ultimately contributing to the cell's propensity to undergo apoptotic death under stressful conditions (12, 13). Most of the work defining the biochemical consequences of mtDNA LHON mutation was done initially taking advantage of *ex-vivo* biological samples from patients, such as platelets, fibroblasts and muscle biopsies, and exploiting the cybrid cell model (4, 14). More recently, a mouse model carrying the ortholog of a rare human pathogenic variant of LHON became available and studies on this model supported a prevalent impact of ROS overproduction on cell physiology, recapitulating some LHON features at histopathology (15).

4.2. Complex I dysfunction impacts cell physiology of retinal ganglion cells

Recently, integrated cell studies including cybrids, fibroblasts and iPSC-derived neurons, demonstrated how the global mitochondrial homeostatic control may be broken by the LHON mtDNA pathogenic variants (16). The mitochondrial life cycle is regulated by mitochondrial dynamics, through continuous fission and fusion events (17) adapting to the needs of cell metabolism (18), and which are strictly instrumental to maintenance of the mitochondrial network mediating between mitochondrial biogenesis and mitochondrial removal through the quality control process of mitochondrial autophagy, namely "mitophagy" (19). Thus, evidence has accumulated that LHON mtDNA pathogenic variants evoke a compensatory activation of mitochondrial biogenesis (20, 21), and that this is an effective cellular strategy to counteract mitochondrial dysfunction (22).There is also, on the other end of the homeostatic process, increasing evidence that mitochondrial dysfunction may activate pathologic mitophagy to levels overwhelming the physiological quality control program (16, 23). Excessive mitophagy may ultimately trigger apoptosis (24) and is driven by the mtDNA LHON pathogenic variant, as this phenotype is transferred with mtDNA into cybrids, which lack the patient's original nuclear DNA (16). It has been proposed that in unaffected carriers of LHON there is an efficient activation of mitochondrial biogenesis that counterbalances the pathologic mitophagy. This reaches a homeostatic balance between the two processes, whereas in those individuals who undergo visual loss, becoming affected with LHON, the mitochondrial biogenesis is not activated enough to reach this compensation (16). This may explain some of the variable penetrance of LHON from a mechanistic point of view (16, 20). In this framework, the high estrogen levels in females, which promote, through the estrogen receptor beta, mitochondrial biogenesis, may also explain the observed male prevalence in LHON (25). Environmental exposure to toxins, like tobacco smoking, which has been shown to hamper mitochondrial biogenesis (26), may further explain the impact of environment on LHON penetrance (27, 28). It must be considered that other interpretations challenge this mechanistic paradigm that emphasizes mitophagy (29), as well as mitochondrial bioenergetics (30) in LHON. Notwithstanding these critical views, observations on activated mitochondrial biogenesis and excessive mitophagy have been obtained by a variety of models, including iPSCs-derived neurons (16), as well as *ex-vivo* tissue samples such as muscle biopsies (20). Also supportive have been the analysis of rare post-mortem retinal specimens from LHON affected and unaffected mutation carrier individuals (16, 20). Remarkably, increased mitophagy seems to lead to deleterious consequences in retinal ganglion cells, as exemplified by experimental work in another mitochondrial optic neuropathy, dominant optic atrophy (DOA) due to mutations in the OPA1 fusion protein (31-33). The specific vulnerability of retinal ganglion cells (RGCs) and their axons as opposed to other neuronal systems represents the next layer in the unravelling pathophysiology of LHON (34).

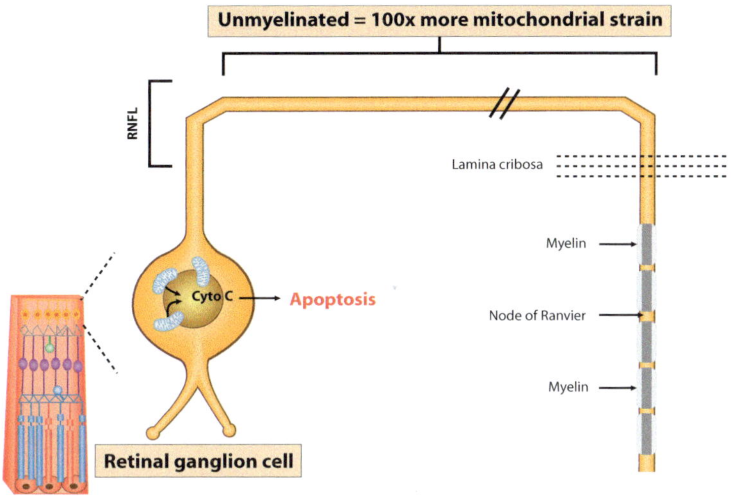

Figure 4.2: The Retinal Ganglion Cell (RGC) is very vulnerable to mitochondrial impairment. Like other neurons, it consumes a great deal of ATP to re-establish its membrane potential after every axon potential. It does not benefit from the metabolic economy of myelin. The RNFL is unmyelinated due to the need for retinal optical transparency, creating a great deal of extra metabolic strain. Adapted from ref. (3).

4.3. The specific vulnerability of RGCs and their axons

Why are axons of the central nervous system so vulnerable to mitochondrial dysfunctions? Most particularly, why is the optic nerve and especially the small axons that constitute the papillo-macular bundle (PMB) so vulnerable? As Figure 4.2 shows, the RGC contributes a long non-myelinated axon that, with the other 1.2 million axons constitutes the retinal nerve fiber layer (RNFL) (4, 34). These fibers must remain unmyelinated as in occupying the most superficial layer of the retina, they must remain transparent to light that passes through them to reach the more posteriorly located rods and cones that transduce light into membrane potentials. Lacking myelin makes the RGC's axons particularly vulnerable to mitochondrial dysfunctions as they have many orders of magnitude more exposed membrane to repolarize after each action potential (35). It is only posterior to the lamina cribrosa, where myelin starts, that saltatory conduction and better energy economy begins (4, 34). This repolarization of the PMB in the retina requires large amounts of ATP supported by mitochondrial respiration, which, in turn, generates lots of ROS. In the presence of LHON pathogenic variants, the complex I dysfunction increases ROS and the aforementioned imbalance of mitochondrial homeostatic control triggers the cascade of deleterious events eventually leading to apoptosis of RGCs and axonal degeneration (4, 16, 20).

In some cases (such as for the *m.3460G>A* variant affecting ND1), the exact mechanism leading from complex I dysfunction to ROS over-production has been worked out (36). These downstream events impinge on the relocation of mitochondria in RGCs, which may get stuck at the emergence of the axonal hillock, as well as the organelle axonal transport which may be profoundly altered (4, 34, 35). So, what happens to the RGCs with an LHON mutation that enhances the over-production of ROS? In a faithful mouse model carrying an ND6 rare mutation associated with LHON in humans (15), the net effect was impaired complex I function, but negligible depletion of ATP and a great over-production of ROS. How does this specifically kill the RGC?

Following each axonal action potential, the sodium/potassium pumps must re-establish the sodium and potassium gradients that create the electrical potential across the axonal membrane; ATP supplies the energy for this pumping. By limiting this process to the small gaps between long stretches of myelin, the Nodes of Ranvier, there is an economy of two to three orders of magnitude (34). However, as just mentioned, RGC axons must remain unmyelinated in the eye, to allow light penetration. RCGs must maintain a high con-

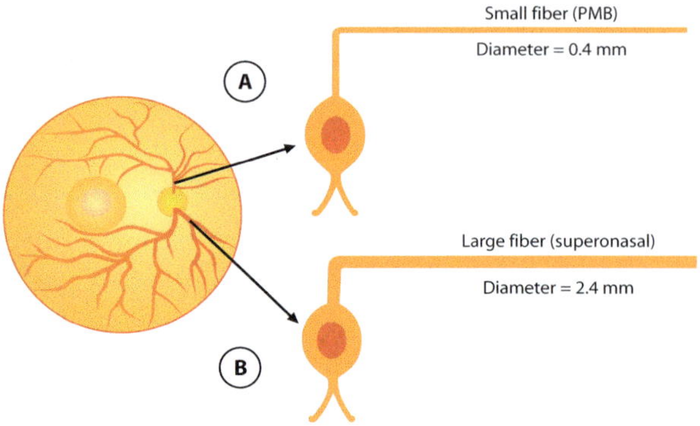

Membrane area to volume ratio

Axon A (small):

$$\frac{\text{Membrane area}}{\text{Volume}} = \frac{L \times 2\pi R}{L \times \pi R^2} = \frac{L(6.28)(0.2)}{L(3.14)(.04)} = \frac{1.26}{0.126} = 10$$

Axon B (large):

$$\frac{\text{Membrane area}}{\text{Volume}} = \frac{L \times 2\pi R}{L \times \pi R^2} = \frac{L(6.28)(1.2)}{L(3.14)(1.44)} = \frac{7.536}{4.52} = 1.67$$

Figure 4.3: Comparison of the metabolic strain in smaller axons that are concentrated in the papillo-macular bundle (PMB). The smaller fiber (**A**) has a diameter of about 0.4 microns. The PMB fiber has a much-reduced volume holding fewer mitochondria. Though its surface area is a little less than a larger fiber, the surface area/volume ratios are six times worse in the smaller fibers, explaining why they are the first to die in LHON. Adapted from ref. (3).

centration of mitochondria to provide this high energy demand and they accumulate, especially in the unmyelinated RNFL and prelaminar portions of the optic nerve head (☞ Figure 4.2). This mitochondrial accumulation provides sufficient ATP for these unmyelinated and highly active fibers, but there is a strain on the system (37).

Collapse of compensation can occur with mitochondrial impairments such as in LHON mtDNA mutations. This is particularly apt to occur to the small fibers of the PMB where high surface to volume ratios makes them particularly vulnerable and, indeed, the PMB fibers are selectively lost early in LHON (☞ Figure 4.3) (38). As these PMB fibers subserve central vision, color vision and high contrast, it's not surprising that these are the presenting characteristics of visual impairment in LHON.

In conclusion, we now have a fairly good understanding of the biochemical features connecting the LHON pathogenic variants to complex I dysfunction, in particular for the *m.3460G>A* variant. Complex I dysfunction may reach a threshold of unbalancing the general homeostasis of mitochondria, including ROS overproduction, mitochondrial membrane potentials and their biogenesis, dynamics and elimination by mitophagy, ultimately impinging on their transport and function in RGCs. The peculiar features of RGC structure and function determines their specific vulnerability, especially for the small axons of the PMB. Each of these steps may provide a therapeutic target, including some current therapies. The manipulation of such dysfunctional steps and pathways enlarges the list of possible therapeutic approaches, leaving LHON at the forefront for cures in mitochondrial medicine.

References

1. Newman NJ, Yu-Wai-Man P, Biousse V, Carelli V. Understanding the molecular basis and pathogenesis of hereditary optic neuropathies: towards improved diagnosis and management. Lancet Neurol. 2023;22(2):172-188.

2. Carroll J, Fearnley IM, Shannon RJ, Hirst J, Walker JE. Analysis of the subunit composition of complex I from bovine heart mitochondria. Mol Cell Proteomics. 2003; 2(2):117-26.

3. Stenton SL, Sheremet NL, Catarino CB, Andreeva NA, Assouline Z, Barboni P, Barel O, Berutti R, Bychkov I, Caporali L, Capristo M, Carbonelli M, Cascavilla ML, Charbel Issa P, Freisinger P, Gerber S, Ghezzi D, Graf E, Heidler J, Hempel M, Heon E, Itkis YS, Javasky E, Kaplan J, Kopajtich R, Kornblum C, Kovacs-Nagy R, Krylova TD, Kunz WS, La Morgia C, Lamperti C, Ludwig C, Malacarne PF, Maresca A, Mayr JA, Meisterknecht J, Nevinitsyna TA, Palombo F, Pode-Shakked B, Shmelkova MS, Strom TM, Tagliavini F, Tzadok M, van der

Ven AT, Vignal-Clermont C, Wagner M, Zakharova EY, Zhorzholadze NV, Rozet JM, Carelli V, Tsygankova PG, Klopstock T, Wittig I, Prokisch H. Impaired complex I repair causes recessive Leber's hereditary optic neuropathy. J Clin Invest. 2021;131(6):e138267.

4. Carelli V, Ross-Cisneros FN, Sadun AA. Mitochondrial dysfunction as a cause of optic neuropathies. Prog Retin Eye Res. 2004;23(1):53-89.

5. Fiedorczuk K, Sazanov LA. Mammalian Mitochondrial Complex I Structure and Disease-Causing Mutations. Trends Cell Biol 2018;28(10):835-867.

6. Carelli V, Ghelli A, Ratta M, Bacchilega E, Sangiorgi S, Mancini R, Leuzzi V, Cortelli P, Montagna P, Lugaresi E, Degli Esposti M. Leber's hereditary optic neuropathy: biochemical effect of 11778/ND4 and 3460/ND1 mutations and correlation with the mitochondrial genotype. Neurology 1997;48(6):1623-32.

7. Carelli V, Ghelli A, Bucchi L, Montagna P, De Negri A, Leuzzi V, Carducci C, Lenaz G, Lugaresi E, Degli Esposti M. Biochemical features of mtDNA 14484 (ND6/M64V) point mutation associated with Leber's hereditary optic neuropathy. Ann Neurol 1999;45:320-8.

8. Hofhaus G, Johns DR, Hurko O, Attardi G, Chomyn A. Respiration and growth defects in transmitochondrial cell lines carrying the 11778 mutation associated with Leber's hereditary optic neuropathy. J Biol Chem. 1996; 271(22):13155-61.

9. Baracca A, Solaini G, Sgarbi G, Lenaz G, Baruzzi A, Schapira AH, Martinuzzi A, Carelli V. Severe impairment of complex I-driven adenosine triphosphate synthesis in Leber hereditary optic neuropathy cybrids. Arch Neurol. 2005;62(5):730-6.

10. Beretta S, Mattavelli L, Sala G, Tremolizzo L, Schapira AH, Martinuzzi A, Carelli V, Ferrarese C. Leber hereditary optic neuropathy mtDNA mutations disrupt glutamate transport in cybrid cell lines. Brain. 2004;127(Pt 10):2183-92.

11. Floreani M, Napoli E, Martinuzzi A, Pantano G, De Riva V, Trevisan R, Bisetto E, Valente L, Carelli V, Dabbeni-Sala F. Antioxidant defences in cybrids harboring mtDNA mutations associated with Leber's hereditary optic neuropathy. FEBS J. 2005;272(5):1124-35.

12. Danielson SR, Wong A, Carelli V, Martinuzzi A, Schapira AH, Cortopassi GA. Cells bearing mutations causing Leber's hereditary optic neuropathy are sensitized to Fas-Induced apoptosis. J Biol Chem. 2002; 277(8):5810-5.

13. Ghelli A, Zanna C, Porcelli AM, Schapira AH, Martinuzzi A, Carelli V, Rugolo M. Leber's hereditary optic neuropathy (LHON) pathogenic mutations induce mitochondrial-dependent apoptotic death in transmitochondrial cells incubated with galactose medium. J Biol Chem. 2003;278(6):4145-50.

14. Carelli V, Rugolo M, Sgarbi G, Ghelli A, Zanna C, Baracca A, Lenaz G, Napoli E, Martinuzzi A, Solaini G. Bioenergetics shapes cellular death pathways in Leber's hereditary optic neuropathy: a model of mitochondrial neurodegeneration. Biochim Biophys Acta. 2004; 1658(1-2):172-9.

15. Chun Shi Lin, Mark S Sharpley, Weiwei Fan, Katrina G Waymire, Alfredo A Sadun, Valerio Carelli, Fred N Ross-Cisneros, Peter Baciu, Eric Sung, Meagan J McManus, Billy X Pan, Daniel W Gil, Grant R Macgregor, Douglas C Wallace. Mouse mtDNA mutant model of Leber hereditary optic neuropathy. Proc Natl Acad Sci U S A. 2012;109(49):20065-70.

16. Danese A, Patergnani S, Maresca A, Peron C, Raimondi A, Caporali L, Marchi S, La Morgia C, Del Dotto V, Zanna C, Iannielli A, Segnali A, Di Meo I, Cavaliere A, Lebiedzinska-Arciszewska M, Wieckowski MR, Martinuzzi A, Moraes-Filho MN, Salomao SR, Berezovsky A, Belfort R Jr, Buser C, Ross-Cisneros FN, Sadun AA, Tacchetti C, Broccoli V, Giorgi C, Tiranti V, Carelli V, Pinton P. Pathological mitophagy disrupts mitochondrial homeostasis in Leber's hereditary optic neuropathy. Cell Rep. 2022;40(3):111124.

17. Chan DC. Mitochondrial Dynamics and Its Involvement in Disease. Annu Rev Pathol. 2020;15:235-259.

18. Mishra P, Carelli V, Manfredi G, Chan DC. Proteolytic cleavage of Opa1 stimulates mitochondrial inner membrane fusion and couples fusion to oxidative phosphorylation. Cell Metab. 2014;19(4):630-41.

19. Twig G, Shirihai OS. The interplay between mitochondrial dynamics and mitophagy. Antioxid Redox Signal. 2011;14(10):1939-51.

20. Giordano C, Iommarini L, Giordano L, Maresca A, Pisano A, Valentino ML, Caporali L, Liguori R, Deceglie S, Roberti M, Fanelli F, Fracasso F, Ross-Cisneros FN, D'Adamo P, Hudson G, Pyle A, Yu-Wai-Man P, Chinnery PF, Zeviani M, Salomao SR, Berezovsky A, Belfort R Jr, Ventura DF, Moraes M, Moraes Filho M, Barboni P, Sadun F, De Negri A, Sadun AA, Tancredi A, Mancini M, d'Amati G, Loguercio Polosa P, Cantatore P, Carelli V. Efficient mitochondrial biogenesis drives incomplete penetrance in Leber's hereditary optic neuropathy. Brain 2014;137(Pt 2):335-53.

21. Bianco A, Martínez-Romero I, Bisceglia L, D'Agruma L, Favia P, Ruiz-Pesini E, Guerriero S, Montoya J, Petruzzella V. Mitochondrial DNA copy number differentiates the Leber's hereditary optic neuropathy affected individuals from the unaffected mutation carriers. Brain. 2016;139(Pt 1):e1.

22. Filograna R, Mennuni M, Alsina D, Larsson NG. Mitochondrial DNA copy number in human disease: the more the better? FEBS Lett. 2021;595(8):976-1002.

23. Dombi E, Diot A, Morten K, Carver J, Lodge T, Fratter C, Ng YS, Liao C, Muir R, Blakely EL, Hargreaves I, Al-Dosary M, Sarkar G, Hickman SJ, Downes SM, Jayawant S, Yu-Wai-Man P, Taylor RW, Poulton J. The m.13051G>A mitochondrial DNA mutation results in variable neurology and activated mitophagy. Neurology. 2016;86(20):1921-3.

24. Bialik S, Dasari SK, Kimchi A. Autophagy-dependent cell death - where, how and why a cell eats itself to death. J Cell Sci. 2018;131(18):jcs215152.

25. Giordano C, Montopoli M, Perli E, Orlandi M, Fantin M, Ross-Cisneros FN, Caparrotta L, Martinuzzi A, Ragazzi E, Ghelli A, Sadun AA, d'Amati G, Carelli V. Oestrogens ameliorate mitochondrial dysfunction in Leber's hereditary optic neuropathy. Brain. 2011;134(Pt 1):220-34.

26. Giordano L, Deceglie S, d'Adamo P, Valentino ML, La Morgia C, Fracasso F, Roberti M, Cappellari M, Petrosillo G, Ciaravolo S, Parente D, Giordano C, Maresca A, Iommarini L, Del Dotto V, Ghelli AM, Salomao SR, Berezovsky A, Belfort R Jr, Sadun AA, Carelli V, Loguercio Polosa P, Cantatore P. Cigarette toxicity triggers Leber's hereditary optic neuropathy by affecting mtDNA copy number, oxidative phosphorylation and ROS detoxification pathways. Cell Death Dis. 2015;6(12):e2021.

27. Kirkman MA, Yu-Wai-Man P, Korsten A, Leonhardt M, Dimitriadis K, De Coo IF, Klopstock T, Chinnery PF. Gene-environment interactions in Leber hereditary optic neuropathy. Brain. 2009;132(Pt 9):2317-26.

28. Carelli V, d'Adamo P, Valentino ML, La Morgia C, Ross-Cisneros FN, Caporali L, Maresca A, Loguercio Polosa P, Barboni P, De Negri A, Sadun F, Karanjia R, Salomao SR, Berezovsky A, Chicani F, Moraes M, Moraes Filho M, Belfort R Jr, Sadun AA. Parsing the differences in affected with LHON: genetic versus environmental triggers of disease conversion. Brain. 2016;139(Pt 3):e17.

29. Sharma LK, Tiwari M, Rai NK, Bai Y. Mitophagy activation repairs Leber's hereditary optic neuropathy-associated mitochondrial dysfunction and improves cell survival. Hum Mol Genet. 2019;28(3):422-433.

30. Lopez Sanchez MIG, Van Bergen NJ, Kearns LS, Ziemann M, Liang H, Hewitt AW, Mackey DA, Trounce IA. OXPHOS bioenergetic compensation does not explain disease penetrance in Leber hereditary optic neuropathy. Mitochondrion. 2020;54:113-121.

31. Liao C, Ashley N, Diot A, Morten K, Phadwal K, Williams A, Fearnley I, Rosser L, Lowndes J, Fratter C, Ferguson DJ, Vay L, Quaghebeur G, Moroni I, Bianchi S, Lamperti C, Downes SM, Sitarz KS, Flannery PJ, Carver J, Dombi E, East D, Laura M, Reilly MM, Mortiboys H, Prevo R, Campanella M, Daniels MJ, Zeviani M, Yu-Wai-Man P, Simon AK, Votruba M, Poulton J. Dysregulated mitophagy and mitochondrial organization in optic atrophy due to OPA1 mutations. Neurology 2017; 88(2):131-142.

32. Carelli V, Musumeci O, Caporali L, Zanna C, La Morgia C, Del Dotto V, Porcelli AM, Rugolo M, Valentino ML, Iommarini L, Maresca A, Barboni P, Carbonelli M, Trombetta C, Valente EM, Patergnani S, Giorgi C, Pinton P, Rizzo G, Tonon C, Lodi R, Avoni P, Liguori R, Baruzzi A, Toscano A, Zeviani M. Syndromic parkinsonism and dementia associated with OPA1 missense mutations. Ann Neurol. 2015;78(1):21-38.

33. Zaninello M, Palikaras K, Naon D, Iwata K, Herkenne S, Quintana-Cabrera R, Semenzato M, Grespi F, Ross-Cisneros FN, Carelli V, Sadun AA, Tavernarakis N, Scorrano L. Inhibition of autophagy curtails visual loss in a model of autosomal dominant optic atrophy. Nat Commun. 2020;11(1):4029.

34. Spiegel SJ and Sadun AA. Int Solutions to a Radical Problem: Overview of Current andFuture Treatment Strategies in Leber's Hereditary Optic Neuropathy. J Mol Sci 2022, 23, 13205.

35. Carelli V, La Morgia C, Ross-Cisneros FN, Sadun AA. Optic neuropathies: the tip of the neurodegeneration iceberg. Hum Mol Genet. 2017;26(R2):R139-R150.

36. Fuller JT 3rd, Barnes S, Sadun LA, Ajmera P, Alexandrova AN, Sadun AA. Coenzyme Q10 trapping in mitochondrial complex I underlies Leber's hereditary optic neuropathy. Proc Natl Acad Sci U S A. 2023 Sep 26;120(39).

37. Pan BX, Ross-Cisneros FN, Carelli V, Rue KS, Salomao SR, Moraes-Filho MN, Moraes MN, Berezovsky A, Belfort R Jr, Sadun AA. Mathematically modeling the involvement of axons in Leber's hereditary optic neuropathy. Invest Ophthalmol Vis Sci. 2012;53:7608-17.

38. Sadun AA, Win PH, Ross-Cisneros FN, Walker SO, Carelli V. Leber's hereditary optic neuropathy differentially affects smaller axons in the optic nerve. Trans Am Ophthalmol Soc. 2000;98:223-32; discussion 232-5.

5. Phenotypes of LHON

Claudia Priglinger, Piero Barboni

LHON typically is perceived as a disease of young men, who experience acute or subacute painless and progressive vision loss in one eye, followed by similar symptoms in the other eye two or three months later. In 25% of cases, visual loss is bilateral at onset and in the majority of the patients both eyes are affected within six months.

At disease onset, affected individuals experience blurring of vision affecting the central visual field due to the early involvement and, later on, degeneration of predominantly retinal ganglion cells (RGC) with smaller caliber fibers in the papillomacular bundle. The small caliber fibers of the papillomacular bundle are selectively lost at a very early stage and the affected eye characteristically demonstrates an early atrophy, while in the arcuate bundles still a pseudoedematous appearance is present.

Because the small fibers transmit foveal and perifoveal color perception, dyschromatopsia is a common sign in the very beginning (1). The most characteristic feature then is an enlarging central scotoma and as the visual field defect increases in size and density, visual acuity deteriorates to the level of counting fingers or worse.

Axonal loss is preceded by a typical swelling of the optic nerve head and pseudopapilledema that then converts into optic disc atrophy worse on the temporal side over a few months. Following nadir, visual acuity may rarely improve and it must be emphasized that the chance for recovery of visual function in LHON is low.

Most patients share the pathognomonic triad of ophthalmological features – as a hallmark – comprising circumpapillary teleangiectatic microangiopathy without leakage on fluorescein angiography and swelling of the retinal nerve fiber layer which allows an ophthalmological diagnosis during the subacute phase. The greater availability of molecular genetic testing has broadened the phenotypical spectrum associated with LHON to include patients with slowly progressive courses with visual deterioration exceeding 6 months, those with insidious or subclinical modes of onset characterized by incidental discovery of subnormal vision and optic atrophy, those with an atypical age at onset, female gender, disease courses associated with neurological disease and only recently LHON with an autosomal recessive (a.r.) mode of inheritance. Therefore, the term "LHON" increasingly is used as a descriptive term for a genetically determined optic neuropathy characterized by painless and, in most cases, permanent loss of central vision in first one eye and then the partner eye in young males. However, the dynamics of the disease and the extent of vision loss, as well as the rates of recovery, are influenced by the underlying causative mutation, the age at onset but also the mode of inheritance.

For this reason, the phenotypic characterization most commonly refers to the clinical stages. Regarding the final visual prognosis, however, LHON-causing pathogenic variants, mode of onset and age at vision loss must be taken into account as influencing factors and slowly progressive courses, childhood-onset disease and late-onset LHON should be considered as distinct clinical variants. The present chapter focuses on maternally inherited LHON (for arLHON ☞ Chapter 8.).

LHON phenotypes	
1.	Typical clinical course
1.1.	Asymptomatic
1.2.	Subacute stage (<6 months from onset)
1.3.	Dynamic stage (6-12 months from onset)
1.4.	Chronic stage (>12 months from onset)
2.	Atypical LHON
2.1	Childhood onset (onset at <12 years)
2.2	Late-onset (onset at >50 years)
2.3	LHON plus
2.4	Atypical clinical course (insidious, unilateral, subclinical, slowly progressive)

5.1. Clinical course of adult-onset LHON

According to the international consensus statement on the clinical and therapeutic management of LHON from 2016, LHON is categorized into four distinct clinical stages (2):

- Asymptomatic mutation carriers
- Subacute LHON (<6 months from onset)
- Dynamic LHON (6-12 months)
- Chronic LHON (>12 months).

5.1.1. Asymptomatic LHON

Asymptomatic carriers of mtDNA pathogenic variants have no identifiable deficiencies in visual performances in standard clinical examinations. Fundus abnormalities including peripapillary telangiectatic vessels and variable degrees of retinal nerve fiber layer pseudoedema can be found and these can vary with time (3) (☞ Figure 5.1).

Using optical coherence tomography (OCT) imaging, thickening of the temporal retinal nerve fiber layer can be confirmed in subgroups of clinically unaffected individuals with a LHON-causing mtDNA pathogenic variant, providing evidence that the papillomacular bundle is particularly vulnerable in LHON (4). On more detailed investigation, some individuals with a LHON-causing mtDNA pathogenic variant can also exhibit subtle impairment of optic nerve function including loss of color vision affecting mostly the red-green system, reduced contrast sensitivity, and subnormal electroretinogram and visual evoked potential (1):

In a large pedigree analysis in Brazil, which included 75 carriers of the m.11778G>A variant, all carriers specifically denied problems with visual acuity, visual field, and color vision. Upon more detailed ophthalmological examination, however, microangiopathy of the optic disc was seen in 21% of the subjects and focal nerve fiber swelling was also seen in 21%. In OCT this swelling corresponded to RNFL thickening of the arcuate bundles. At the functional level, the optic nerve head component was below normal or even missing in multifocal electroretinograms and in many LHON carriers this corresponded with areas of relative paracentral or arcuate scotomas. Tritan defects were found in 40% and deutan defects in 56% of asymptomatic carriers with the m.11778G>A mutation employing the Farnsworth-Munsell 100

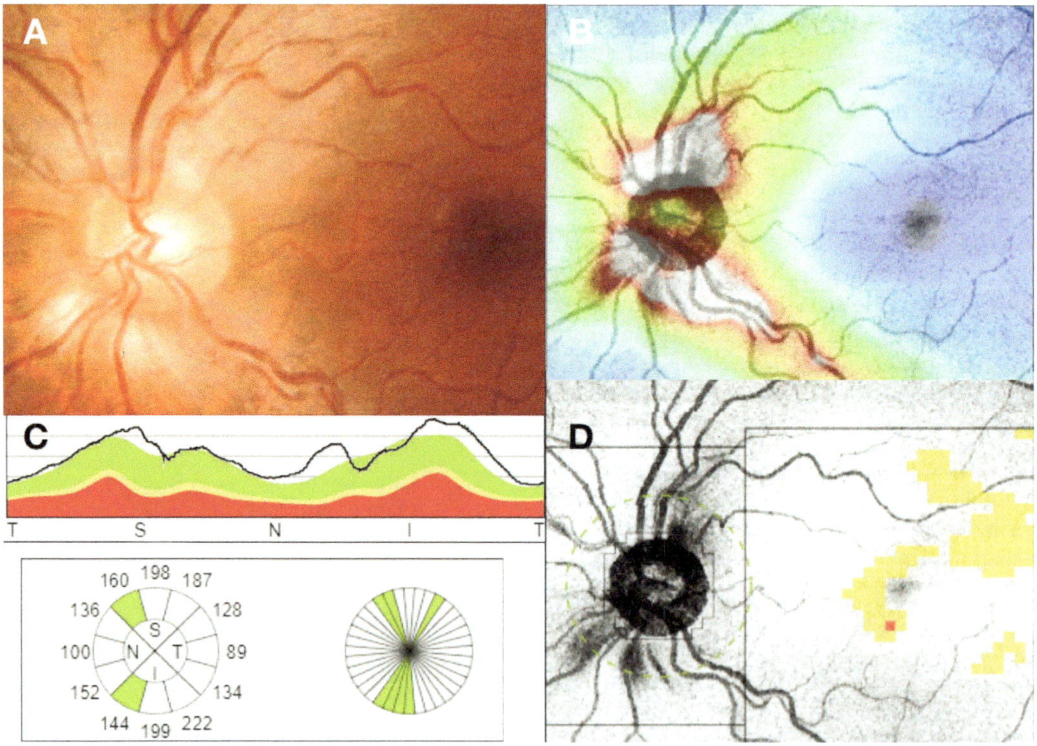

Figure 5.1: Asymptomatic mutation carrier.
A: Fundus picture showing microangiopathy, vessel tortuosity and peripapillary fiber swelling. **B**: RNFL thickness map, **C**: Circular RNFL thickness and GCL thickness map detecting the fiber swelling without RGC damage.

hue test. Although many carriers clearly show presymptomatic signs, this is not predictive for an impending conversion to the subacute stage. To this date, no clinical parameters clearly suggestive of a threatening onset of the disease have been established.

5.1.2. Subacute stage of LHON

The subacute mode of onset is most common. In adults 60 % of patients with the m.11778G>A variant and 40% of patients with the m.3460G>A variant reported a subacute onset of the disease (3). Affected individuals develop blurring of vision affecting the central visual field in one eye and progressive red-green dyschromatopsia. Similar symptoms appear in the other eye two or three months later. The most characteristic feature is an enlarging central scotoma and a severe loss of visual acuity that deteriorates to the level of counting fingers or worse. Even if the central scotoma is the most frequent visual field defect, any other kind of visual field damage can be evident as blind spot enlargement, bitemporal incomplete hemianopia, altitudinal defect and so on (5). Following nadir, visual acuity may rarely improve. In the majority of the patients both eyes are affected within six months and in 25% of cases, visual loss is bilateral at onset (6).

Clinically, optic disc hyperemia, pseudoedema of the peripapillary retinal nerve fiber layer, increased vascular tortuosity and teleangiectasia, as well as temporal optic disc pallor are hallmarks in the subacute phase of vision loss, while these features are absent in 20% (5). About half of the individuals have a swollen or whitish appearance of the nerve fiber layer. A subset of patients even develops peripapillary hemorrhages (3).

Characteristically, in fluorescein angiography there is a lack of exudation from the dilated vessels, but measures of mean tissue perfusion using laser speckle fluorography point at a 32% and 15% higher perfusion in the early subacute stage of the disease, with a subsequent decline in the late subacute and dynamic stage. RNFL thickness as measured by SD-OCT follows a specific pattern of swelling and subsequent atrophy starting from the inferotemporal sectors and followed by superior and nasal sectors. The inferotemporal sector damage corresponding to the papillomacular bundle represent the structural hallmark of the disease conversion which precedes the RGCs damage (7-9) (☞ Figure 5.2A).

5.1.3. Dynamic stage of LHON

In the dynamic stage, we can detect a progressive thinning of RNFL and complete atrophy of RGCs. During the first 6 months after disease onset, the RNFL increase in thickness is followed by progressive thinning until 12 months, maintaining the order of the infero-temporal sectors before and the supero-nasal after. RGCs thinning begins right away after disease onset and reaches the thinnest point at 3-6 months (10).

5.1.4. Chronic stage of LHON

Twelve months after onset LHON typically enters the chronic phase. If untreated, visual acuity has reached a nadir at a mean VA of 0.02 decimal or worse in patients with the m.11778G>A variant. At this stage, 92% of patients have severe dyschromatopsia (3). The optic disc is pale and atrophic with diffuse loss of retinal nerve fibers, while the temporal portion of the optic disc is most affected. In patients with a milder course of the disease, peripapillary microangiopathy still can be present (☞ Figure 5.2B). The central scotoma can further enlarge, but in some patients fenestration can occur.

Visual outcomes in the chronic phase with respect to the underlying pathogenic mitochondrial variant

Recovery of vision in LHON, if it does occur, usually is incomplete and not before 15-18 months from onset. Recovery of vision is defined as improvement of visual field with or without improvement of visual acuity. The central scotoma may be reduced or fenestrated or both. While ganglion cell dysfunction and disease course in the first 12 months appear to follow a rather uniform pattern, probability and extent of improvement depend on the underlying pathogenic LHON mutation, but also on the extent of vision loss at nadir. Favorable prognostic factors are considered: childhood onset, 14484/ND6 mtDNA mutation, larger ONH size. Whereas, as negative prognostic factors are considered: late age at onset and monocular childhood onset, 3460/ND1 mtDNA mutation, smaller ONH size. Reported visual recovery rates for the

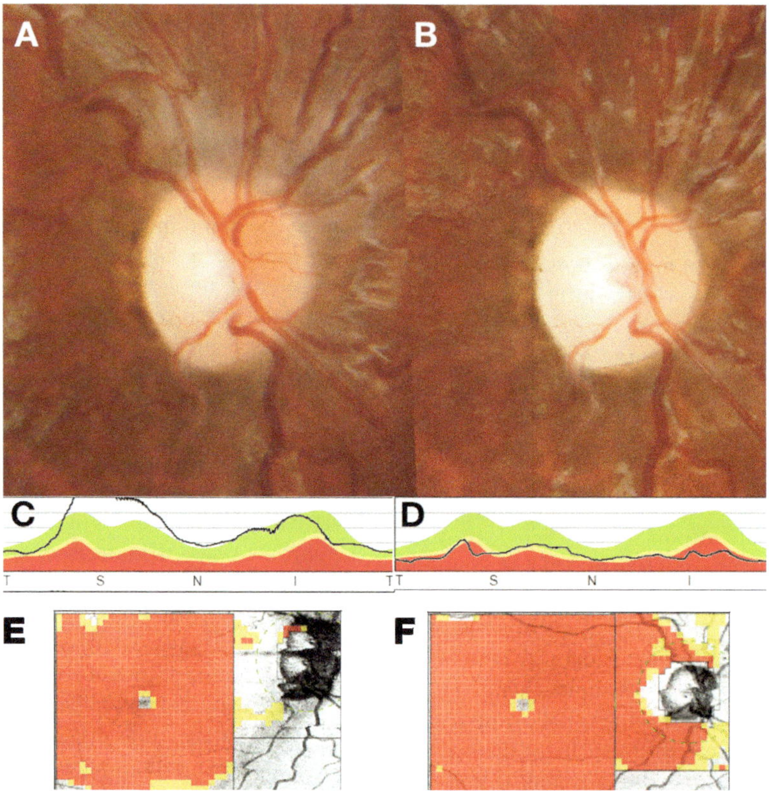

Figure 5.2: Affected patient.
A: Fundus picture 3 months from onset showing swelling of fibers, microangiopathy and temporal pallor of the optic disc. **B**: One year later the optic nerve show diffuse pallor with fiber swelling reduction and vessel straightening and caliper reduction. **C, D**: Peripapillary RNFL thickness, and **E, F**: GCL thickness map showing the early thinning of temporal fibers and ganglion cells and the superior and inferior thickening of fibers at 6 months followed by thinning at 1 year from onset.

major pathogenic LHON mutations are discussed in detail in Chapter 6.

5.2. Atypical LHON

5.2.1. Childhood onset LHON

Childhood LHON is defined by the onset of visual loss under 12 years of age (2), encompassing about 10% of all LHON cases (11-13). Childhood disease has clinical presentation characteristics that distinguish it from the adult form such as a better visual prognosis and more frequent atypical clinical features. Based on the pattern of visual loss, patients can be stratified as subacute bilateral (similar to the classical adult form), insidious bilateral, unilateral, subclinical and slowly progressive (14). When the onset of visual loss is not well defined before 3 years of age it is called insidious, with a frequency of 17% of childhood cases.

Children with bilateral onset before 9 years of age have in general better visual prognosis compared with classical adult LHON. Whereas, unilateral cases have the worst visual prognosis due to the early age at onset and the appearance of strabismus. The second eye in the unilateral cases can remain unaffected or have subclinical involvement or develop visual loss in adult age. Noteworthy, the pedigree analysis showed a familial recurrence of childhood cases of about 17% and a female preponderance in some pedigrees (5, 14).

The relative frequencies of mtDNA mutations in childhood was highest for m.11778G>A (55%) followed by m.14484T>C (23%) and m.3460G>A (17%). The male to female ratio for the childhood onset was 2.9:1.The diagnosis of LHON should be taken into account in children with unexplained low vision also with associated strabismus, in order to avoid a mistake and delay in diagnosis.

5.2.2. Late-onset LHON

Several case reports describe LHON-related vision loss after the age of 50 years. A retrospective cohort analysis identified LHON with late onset in 8% of the patients with a male to female ratio of 3:1. The m.11778G>A mutation was most prevalent (m.11778, 80%; m.3460G>A, 21%; m.14484 T>C, 13%) and subacute loss of central vision like in typical LHON was reported in most cases (14). If patients with late-onset LHON are only examined during the chronic phase, it may be difficult to identify the cause of optic atrophy, particularly if there is no maternal family history of LHON or if they did not encounter the subacute painless sequential bilateral loss of vision.

Numerous environmental factors have been hypothesized to trigger subacute late-onset visual loss in LHON carriers, including trauma, anemia, vitamin B12 deficiency, HIV-medications, smoking and alcohol consumption (15-20). In a cross-sectional analysis of 20 late-onset patients, the lifetime cumulative smoking and alcohol consumption was higher in late onset compared to typical LHON (23.4 versus 4.9 pack years), which is rather self-evident. However, there was no significant difference with regards to daily tobacco and weekly alcohol consumption. On the other hand, late-onset LHON patients had significantly higher cumulative tobacco consumption compared with unaffected carriers of the same age group (23.4 vs 9.3 pack years), which again supports the hypothesis that tobacco may be a factor triggering the onset of LHON but at the same time other than environmental factors may be responsible for the late manifestation as well (15).

5.2.3. LHON plus and LHON-overlap syndromes

Most patients with LHON develop isolated RGCs/optic nerve involvement. However, a subgroup of patients manifests additional neurological features as part of a "LHON plus" phenotype. This phenotype comprises patients who additionally exhibit ataxia, tremor, dystonia, and/or cardiac conduction defects. Occasionally, these patients also present with demyelinating lesions in their central nervous system and manifest with multiple sclerosis-like illness ("Harding's disease"). Furthermore, overlaps with other mitochondriopathies can occur. These variants are referred to as LHON/MELAS (mitochondrial encephalopathy with lactate acidosis and stroke-like episodes) in adults or LHON/Leigh-overlap syndromes in children (21, 22).

5.2.4. Atypical clinical course

Subclinical LHON

Subclinical LHON refers to patients who are subjectively not aware of a loss of visual function. However, upon ophthalmological examination mild functional damage with VA between 0.8 and 1.0 decimal or a small central or paracentral scotoma together with mild structural pathological changes such as temporal optic disc pallor and temporal RNFL thinning and and/or macular GCL thickness reduction on OCT can be revealed. These cases have been suggested to denote an abortive onset, which did not progress to the anatomical threshold of RGC loss that would result in symptomatic visual deterioration. This situation can be found in some presumably asymptomatic carriers as well as in unilateral courses, where one eye is severely affected while the partner eye has only subclinical signs of LHON (3, 14).

Slowly progressive LHON

Slowly progressive LHON is a rather rare phenotypical presentation and is defined as a progressive vision loss over more than 6 months. In a retrospective analysis, this mode of onset was rare in adults (4%), but occurred in 15% of children with LHON. In a first case series from 2006, a slowly progressive course after childhood onset accounted for a favorable visual outcome with a mean VA of 0.4-0.6 decimal (3, 12, 13).

References

1. Sadun AA, Salomao SR, Berezovsky A, Sadun F, Denegri AM, Quiros PA, et al. Subclinical carriers and conversions in Leber hereditary optic neuropathy: a prospective psychophysical study. Transactions of the American Ophthalmological Society. 2006;104:51-61.

2. Carelli V, Carbonelli M, de Coo IF, Kawasaki A, Klopstock T, Lagreze WA, et al. International consensus statement on the clinical and therapeutic management of Leber Hereditary Optic Neuropathy. Journal of Neuro-Ophthalmology. 2017;37(4):371-81.

3. Nikoskelainen EK, Huoponen K, Juvonen V, Lamminen T, Nummelin K, Savontaus ML. Ophthalmologic findings in Leber hereditary optic neuropathy, with special reference to mtDNA mutations. Ophthalmology. 1996;103(3):504-14.

4. Savini G, Barboni P, Valentino ML, Montagna P, Cortelli P, De Negri AM, et al. Retinal nerve fiber layer evaluation by optical coherence tomography in unaffected carriers with Leber's hereditary optic neuropathy mutations. Ophthalmology. 2005;112(1):127-31.

5. Barboni P. Sadun AA. Atlas of LHON. Breukelen, Netherlands: MEDonline; 2019

6. Yu-Wai-Man P, Griffiths PG, Howell N, Turnbull DM, Chinnery PF. The epidemiology of leber hereditary optic neuropathy in the North East of England. Am J Hum Genet. 2016;98(6):1271.

7. Calzetti G, La Morgia C, Cattaneo M, Carta A, Bosello F, Amore G, et al. Longitudinal study of optic disk perfusion and retinal structure in Leber's hereditary optic neuropathy. Invest Ophthalmol Vis Sci. 2022;63(1):43.

8. Barboni P, Carbonelli M, Savini G, Ramos Cdo V, Carta A, Berezovsky A, et al. Natural history of Leber's hereditary optic neuropathy: longitudinal analysis of the retinal nerve fiber layer by optical coherence tomography. Ophthalmology. 2010;117(3):623-7.

9. Carbonelli M, La Morgia C, Romagnoli M, Amore G, D'Agati P, Valentino ML, et al. Capturing the pattern of transition from carrier to affected in Leber hereditary optic neuropathy. American Journal of Ophthalmology. 2022;241:71-9.

10. Balducci N, Savini G, Cascavilla ML, La Morgia C, Triolo G, Giglio R, et al. Macular nerve fibre and ganglion cell layer changes in acute Leber's hereditary optic neuropathy. Br J Ophthalmol. 2016;100(9):1232-7.

11. Siedlecki J, Koenig S, Catarino C, Schaumberger MM, Schworm B, Priglinger SG, et al. Childhood versus early-teenage onset Leber's hereditary optic neuropathy: visual prognosis and capacity for recovery. Br J Ophthalmol. 2022.

12. Majander A, Bowman R, Poulton J, Antcliff RJ, Reddy MA, Michaelides M, et al. Childhood-onset Leber hereditary optic neuropathy. Br J Ophthalmol. 2017;101(11):1505-9.

13. Barboni P, Savini G, Valentino ML, La Morgia C, Bellusci C, De Negri AM, et al. Leber's hereditary optic neuropathy with childhood onset. Invest Ophthalmol Vis Sci. 2006;47(12):5303-9.

14. Barboni P, La Morgia C, Cascavilla ML, Hong EH, Battista M, Majander A, et al. Childhood-Onset Leber Hereditary Optic Neuropathy - Clinical and Prognostic Insights. American Journal of Ophthalmology. 2022.

15. Dimitriadis K, Leonhardt M, Yu-Wai-Man P, Kirkman MA, Korsten A, De Coo IF, et al. Leber's hereditary optic neuropathy with late disease onset: clinical and molecular characteristics of 20 patients. Orphanet Journal of Rare Diseases. 2014;9:158.

16. Moura-Coelho N, Pinto Proenca R, Tavares Ferreira J, Cunha JP. Late-onset Leber's hereditary optic neuropathy: the role of environmental factors in hereditary diseases. BMJ Case Rep. 2019;12(3):e227977.

17. Zhang X, Meagher S, Han MK, Kattah J. Late-onset Leber's hereditary optic neuropathy with concurrent retinal detachment and retrobulbar visual pathway involvement. Neuroophthalmology. 2022;46(4):248-53.

18. Goyal S, Riordan-Eva P, Coakes RL. Late onset of Leber's hereditary optic neuropathy precipitated by anaemia. Eye (Lond). 2004;18(10):1017-8.

19. Yu-Wai-Man P, Bateman DE, Hudson G, Griffiths PG, Chinnery PF. Leber hereditary optic neuropathy presenting in a 75-year-old man. Journal of Neuro-Ophthalmology. 2008;28(2):155.

20. Dagi LR, Rizzo JFI, Cestari DM. Leber Hereditary Optic Neuropathy in an Octogenarian. Journal of Neuro-Ophthalmology. 2008;28(2):156.

21. Finsterer J, Zarrouk-Mahjoub S. Leber's hereditary optic neuropathy is multiorgan not mono-organ. Clin Ophthalmol. 2016;10:2187-90.

22. Matthews L, Enzinger C, Fazekas F, Rovira A, Ciccarelli O, Dotti MT, et al. MRI in Leber's hereditary optic neuropathy: the relationship to multiple sclerosis. Journal of Neurology, Neurosurgery, and Psychiatry. 2015; 86(5):537-42.

6. Natural history of LHON

Rustum Karanjia, Nancy J. Newman, Catherine Vignal-Clermont

The clinical phenotype of Leber's Hereditary Optic Neuropathy (LHON) was first described by Albrecht von Graefe in 1858 and later expanded upon by Theodor Leber in 1871. In the subsequent century, the pathophysiology of LHON and the genetic basis of the disease remained a mystery (☞ Chapters 2. and 4.) and LHON was purely a clinical diagnosis, the phenotype of which is described in more detail in Chapter 5. In the absence of a confirmatory test, this clinical picture was felt to be characteristic. Vision loss with visual field findings of a central scotoma without peripheral contraction is classical for the disease, which by the later stages progresses such that optic atrophy becomes apparent, starting in the temporal sector and progressing to diffuse atrophy. This clinical description still encompasses the key findings of the LHON phenotype, with a few alterations as we have learned more about this disease.

The most significant change in our understanding of LHON occurred in 1988 when the Wallace laboratory reported the first mitochondrial (m.) variant capable of causing LHON. The m.11778G>A variant in ND4, identified by Wallace's group is the most common cause of LHON worldwide, concerning about 70% of subjects and when coupled with two other variants, m.3460G>A in ND1, and m.14484T>C in ND6, account for about 90% of LHON cases.

6.1. Conversion

Disease onset is defined as when the subject first notices a disturbance in their vision and the conversion is the process of going from the unaffected carrier state to the affected state. The sequential nature of conversion and the division of conversion into a subacute and dynamic phase with the accompanying OCT findings are described in Chapter 5. From a natural history perspective, it is important to note that there are case reports of unilateral disease persisting for years to decades. In some of these case reports conversion was instigated by another disease such as multiple sclerosis-associated optic neuritis. Typically, in over 97% of subjects, however, LHON is a bilateral disease (1).

Clinically, the natural history of conversion is continued visual acuity decline for up to 8 months with an accompanying decrease in central vision and visual field mean deviation (2) (☞ Figure 6.1). One year after symptom onset, the end of the dynamic phase, subjects typically reach a plateau with visual acuity worse than 20/800 in both eyes.

Onset in children accounts for about 10% of cases and onset <12 years of age is typically associated with a milder form of the disease than adult-onset cases (3). The disease in children is subclassified as acute if there is rapid deterioration in vision, reaching a nadir within about 6 months, slowly progressive if it takes more than about 6 months to reach the nadir, and, uniquely in childhood onset, as subclinical or insidious where the subject is unaware of vision loss when optic atrophy or subnormal vision is diagnosed, with clinical stability at subsequent follow-ups (4).

Currently it is not possible to predict which subjects will convert from the carrier to the affected state, although exposure to both environmental factors and certain medications have been identified as potential triggers for conversion. Environmental exposure, in particular smoking, has been found to have a strong consistent association with increased likelihood of vision loss, and a trend towards increased visual failure with heavy alcohol intake has also been reported (12). Medications which target essential mitochondrial function have also been implicated in triggering conversion, in particular antimicrobials which target prokaryotic ribosomes also inhibit mitochondrial ribosomes, which share a common lineage (5). The impacts of these medications on affected individuals have not been established. While there is a theoretical risk of harm from the use of these medications in both carriers and affected individuals, it is important to note that some are used to treat life-threatening infections and their use should be balanced with the risks posed by those infections.

6.2. Natural history of chronic LHON

Optic atrophy is the hallmark for the chronic phase of the disease. The atrophy progresses from the

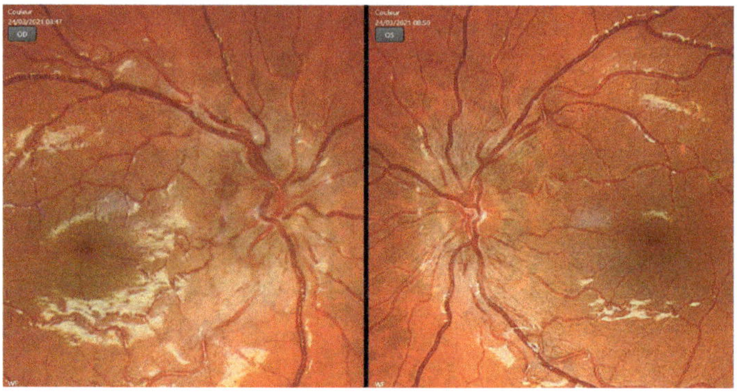

A

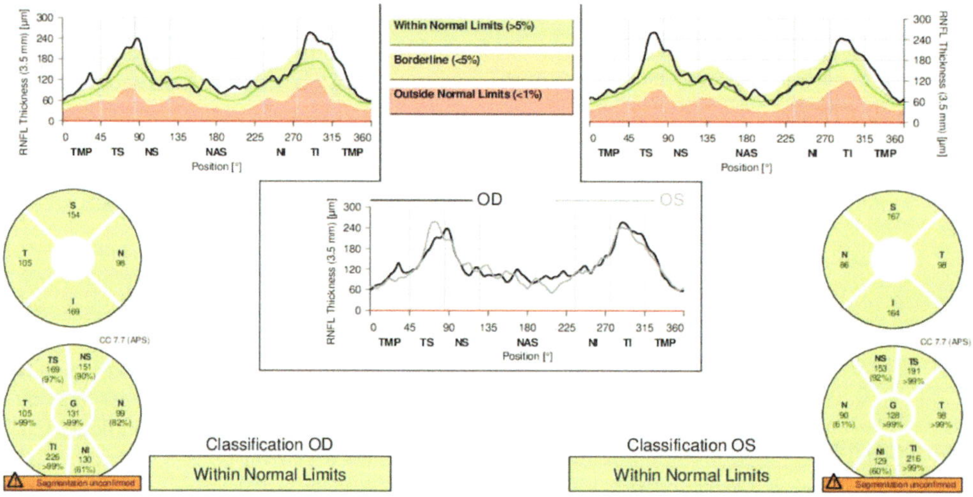
Within Normal Limits (>5%)
Borderline (<5%)
Outside Normal Limits (<1%)
RNFL Thickness (3.5 mm) [µm]
Position [°]
TMP TS NS NAS NI TI TMP
OD
OS
Classification OD
Within Normal Limits
Classification OS
Within Normal Limits
Segmentation unconfirmed

B

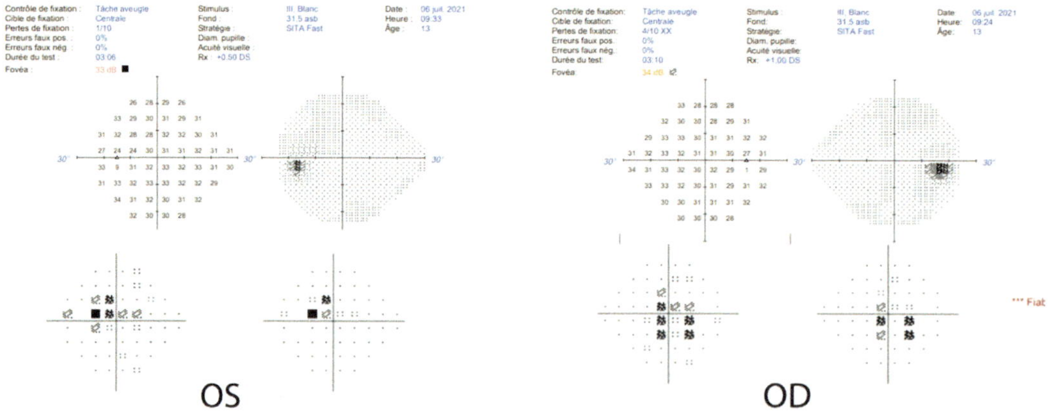
OS
OD

C

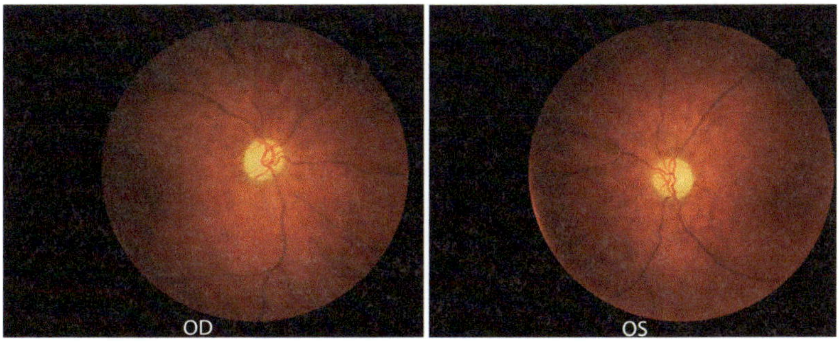

D

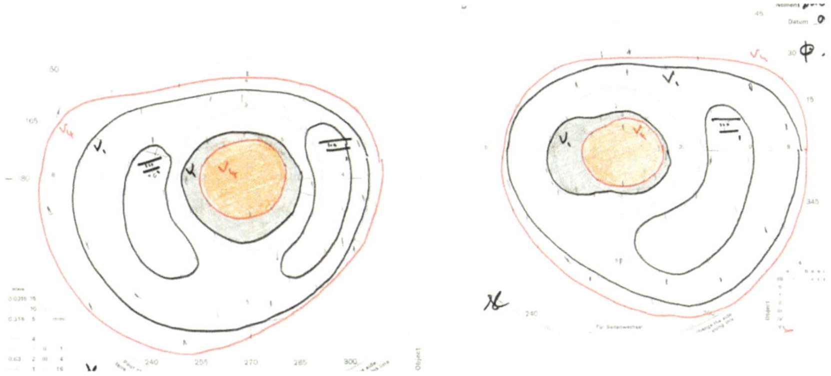

E

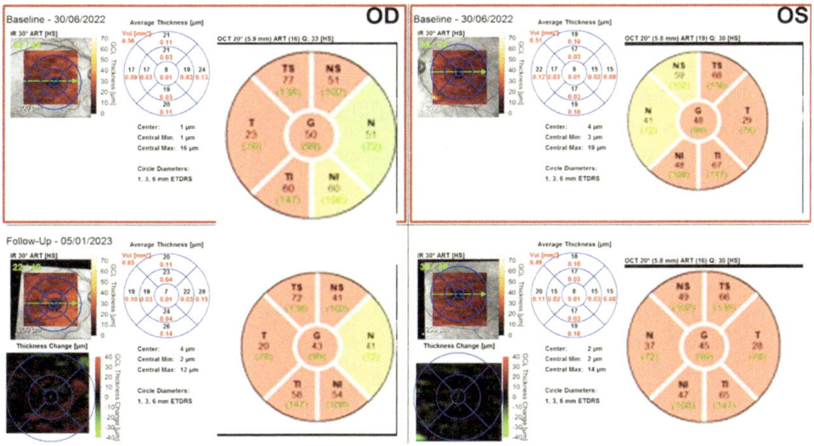

F

Figure 6.1: Conversion and progressive vision loss in a 13-year-old male subject with a family history of LHON with m.11778G>A ND4 variant in a brother and uncle. At age 8 (2016) BCVA 20/20 OU, normal fundus and RNFL thickness of 138 µm OD and 128 µm OS.
A: March 2021 asymptomatic, BCVA 20/20 OU, with new onset optic disc pseudo-edema OU, vascular tortuosity and telangiectasias. **B**: RNFL thickness remains stable at 131 µm OD and 128 µm OS. June 2021 complained of visual disturbance. BCVA decreased to 20/30 OD, 20/40 OS, pseudo-edema and increased thickness of RNFL to 150 µm OD and 152 µm OS. **C**: July 2021 progressive vision loss: BCVA 20/80 OU, Humphrey visual field demonstrating central scotoma and increased RNFL thickness to 160 µm OD and 161 µm OS. **D**: June 2022 and January 2023: BCVA CF 1m OD and 20/800 OS with bilateral optic disc atrophy, bilateral caecocentral scotomas on Goldman Visual Field testing (**E**), and loss of RGC RNFL and macular GCC volume (**F**).

temporal inferior part of the disc to the nasal superior portion, although the rate of progression differs among subjects. As a result, the degree of atrophy can be quite varied, even within the same pedigree (2).

A meta-analysis published in 2020 reports the visual outcome in LHON subjects with the most frequent variant (m.11778G>A variant in ND4, n=695 subjects). Among subjects 15 years and older, recovery of meaningful vision likely occurs in 11.3%, and visual acuities of better than 20/200 are rare. In this paper, an age of onset of less than 12 years portended a better visual prognosis and a different natural history of visual loss progression and recovery than in adults (6). In the same way, a study of Dutch pedigrees found that the mean age of onset of subjects with a visual acuity of 20/200 or worse was 28 years, while among those with a visual acuity of 20/40 or better the mean age of onset was 13 years (7).

A more recent paper reported the natural history of LHON, by a retrospective evaluation of the visual course and outcome of 44 subjects harboring one of the three most common disease-causing mtDNA variants (8). 61% of subjects carried the m.11778G>A variant in ND4, 18% the m.3460G>A in ND1, and 21% the m.14484T>C variant in ND6, with a mean age at onset of 30.2, 24.9, and 23.6 years, respectively. For the entire study cohort, the mean ± standard deviation (SD) best corrected visual acuity (BCVA) was 1.37±0.78 logMAR at the last observed measure i.e., the chronic phase (mean of 32.2 months from onset of vision loss), below 20/200 (1.0 logMAR), the threshold for legal blindness in most countries. Based on the LHON genotype, the BCVA (mean ± SD) was 1.46±0.63 logMAR in m.11778G>A subjects, 1.52±1.06 logMAR in m.3460G>A subjects, and 0.97±0.83 logMAR in m.14484T>C subjects. This data set is complicated by the fact that 57% of these subjects had taken idebenone; yet despite this, 76% of eyes had a BCVA of 1.0 logMAR or worse at last observed measure, >15 years after onset. The proportion of eyes with off-chart BCVA was comparable for the three LHON genotypes (42-48%) but LHON subjects carrying the m.14484T>C variant achieved better final vision compared with those carrying the m.11778G>A and m.3460G>A variants.

Similar findings are reported in a retrospective review of clinical data of patients with genetically confirmed LHON presenting to an Irish tertiary ophthalmic hospital (9). This natural history cohort consisted of 44 patients from 34 pedigrees, 84% male and 75% harboring the m.11778G>A variant. The median review duration was 33.5 months (mean 74.4, range 2.0-431.2 months). As with other studies, the very poor visual prognosis of LHON was reiterated: at final review; mean logMAR BCVA was 1.62±0.76, and legal blindness status (logMAR 1.0 or worse in the better eye) was present in 56.8% of subjects. In this study, preservation of nasal RNFL was the best predictor of on-chart final VA. An age of onset of less than 20 years of age (39% of subjects) also had better VA at the last visit. In contrast, female gender, off-chart visual acuity or optic atrophy at presentation were biomarkers predicting poorer (i.e., 'off-chart') final VA. However, in this cohort, there was no correlation between variant and VA, and mtDNA heteroplasmy was associated with better VA outcomes (0.88 versus 1.76, p=0.092). The authors point out the limitations of this study, which is retrospective, extends over a long period of time and is based on a small sample size.

Combined natural history data from 408 eyes of patients with the m.11778G>A mutation was used as a comparison for a clinical trial treatment group and showed that at the last visit the mean BCVA was 1.68 ± 0.61 with a median follow-up of 25.3 months (0 to 768 months) (10). A LOESS regression model was used to match the data to the clinical trial at 12, 18, 24, 36 and 48 months (☞ Figure 6.2). As most of the natural history data was collected retrospectively, the number of eyes varied between 27 and 80 eyes for each time point. This highlights one of the challenges with retrospective data collection, yet it provides strong evidence that BCVA continues to decline in subjects even after reaching the initial nadir. The majority of eyes of LHON subjects who were below the age of 15 at onset had a BCVA better than 1.0 logMAR at the last observed measure, and all the m.11778G>A and m.14484T>C subjects younger than 15 at onset had on-chart visual acuity in both eyes, confirming the better visual prognosis in these younger groups (8).

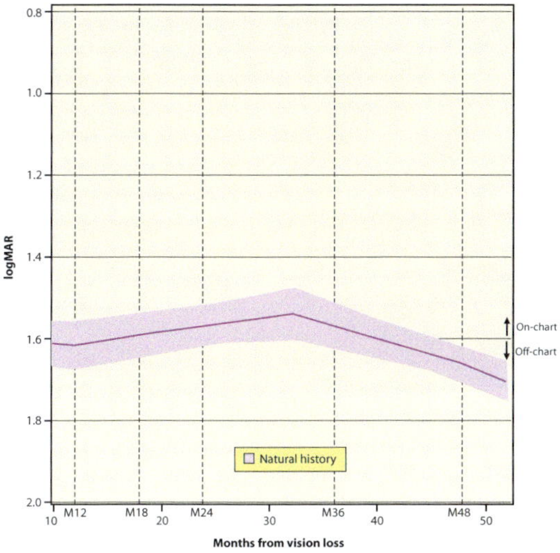

Figure 6.2: Natural history of BCVA in affected subjects with the m.11778G>A variant was estimated by a LOESS regression (solid line) (n=408 eyes) with 95% confidence intervals around the fitted curve (shaded area). Adapted from Carelli et al., 2023, with permission.

6.3. Spontaneous visual recovery

In contrast to the poor vision typically associated with LHON, some subjects experience an untreated partial clinical recovery in vision, termed spontaneous recovery. The clinical cut-off for partial spontaneous recovery varies among publications, showing only a modest one-to-two-line improvement in vision while other case reports list a full recovery to near normal vision. Visual recovery was documented in pedigrees back to the early 1900s; however, some cases were in male descendants on the paternal lineage, suggesting that they were not actually cases of LHON (11). Misdiagnosis is now less likely to occur thanks to the identification of the causative genetic variants, but remains a challenge with incomplete retrospective data.

Partial spontaneous recovery can take two forms, the first is a gradual clearing of the scotoma and return of "normal" Snellen visual acuity while still having scattered decreases in the visual field (☞ Figure 6.3). The second form is a partial clearing of parts of the scotoma such that a small window or fenestration opens in the scotoma which permits the subject to see a small part of the visual field more clearly (☞ Figure 6.4). Subjects can learn to use this fenestration to see by scanning their environment and mentally assembling a more complete picture of the visual field. Subjects who experience spontaneous recovery still experience some visual deficits, particularly with color vision and in low-contrast situations, despite being able to read up to the 20/20 line on a high contrast Snellen eye chart. As in other optic atrophies, normal Snellen visual acuity should not be confused with normal vision.

Rates of spontaneous recovery vary among variants and between studies. This is in part due to considerable variability in how spontaneous recovery is defined and how visual acuity was measured and reported, especially amongst retrospective studies. The time at which subjects were tested is also important, as infrequent testing may miss the true nadir, underestimating recovery rates. There is also an overreliance on visual acuity which only examines the performance of a small portion of the visual angle with a high contrast stimulus.

Amongst the three most common mitochondrial DNA variants, m.14484T>C has the highest reported rate of partial spontaneous recovery between 37% and 71% (12). The recovery rates for the other two primary variants range from 4-23% for m.11778G>A and 15-25% for the m.3460G>A variant (6, 12). Partial spontaneous recovery has also been reported in other genetic variants, but rates of spontaneous recovery are hard to calculate due to small sample sizes. In addition, the widespread use of idebenone confounds the natural history with a potential treatment effect.

Visual outcomes vary among subjects even within the same pedigree and among siblings (13). In a case series of three brothers who were affected by LHON, two siblings had poor visual outcomes while a third had late-onset recovery in vision when he stopped smoking and drinking, suggesting that environmental exposures to mitochondrial toxins may influence spontaneous visual recovery and natural history of the disease. This further confounds natural history data from retrospective studies, as rates of tobacco and alcohol use have changed in societies over the last few decades.

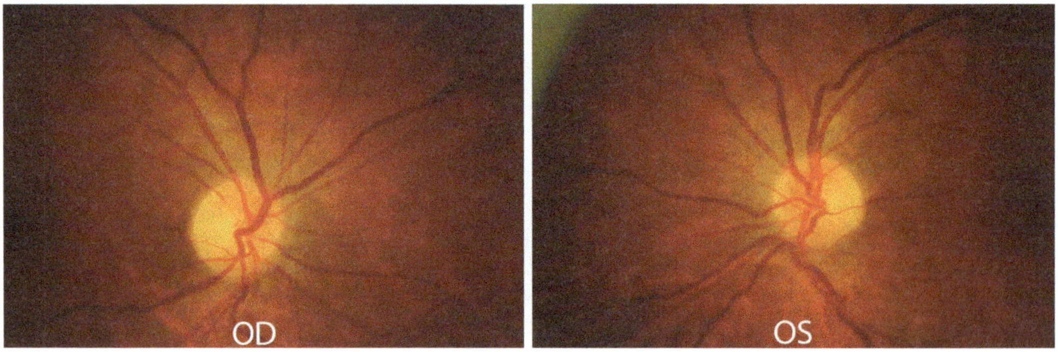
OD
OS

A

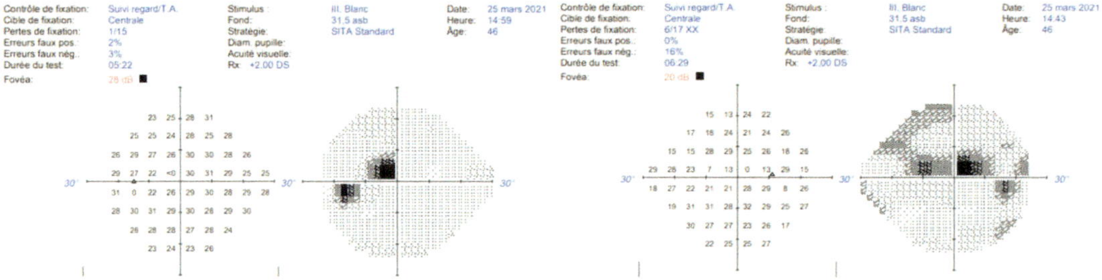
Contrôle de fixation: Suivi regard/T.A.
Cible de fixation: Centrale
Pertes de fixation: 1/15
Erreurs faux pos.: 2%
Erreurs faux nég.: 3%
Durée du test: 05:22
Fovéa: 28 dB
Stimulus: III, Blanc
Fond: 31,5 asb
Stratégie: SITA Standard
Diam. pupille:
Acuité visuelle:
Rx: +2,00 DS
Date: 25 mars 2021
Heure: 14:59
Âge: 46
Contrôle de fixation: Suivi regard/T.A.
Cible de fixation: Centrale
Pertes de fixation: 6/17 XX
Erreurs faux pos.: 0%
Erreurs faux nég.: 16%
Durée du test: 06:29
Fovéa: 20 dB
Stimulus: III, Blanc
Fond: 31,5 asb
Stratégie: SITA Standard
Diam. pupille:
Acuité visuelle:
Rx: +2,00 DS
Date: 25 mars 2021
Heure: 14:43
Âge: 46
30°

B

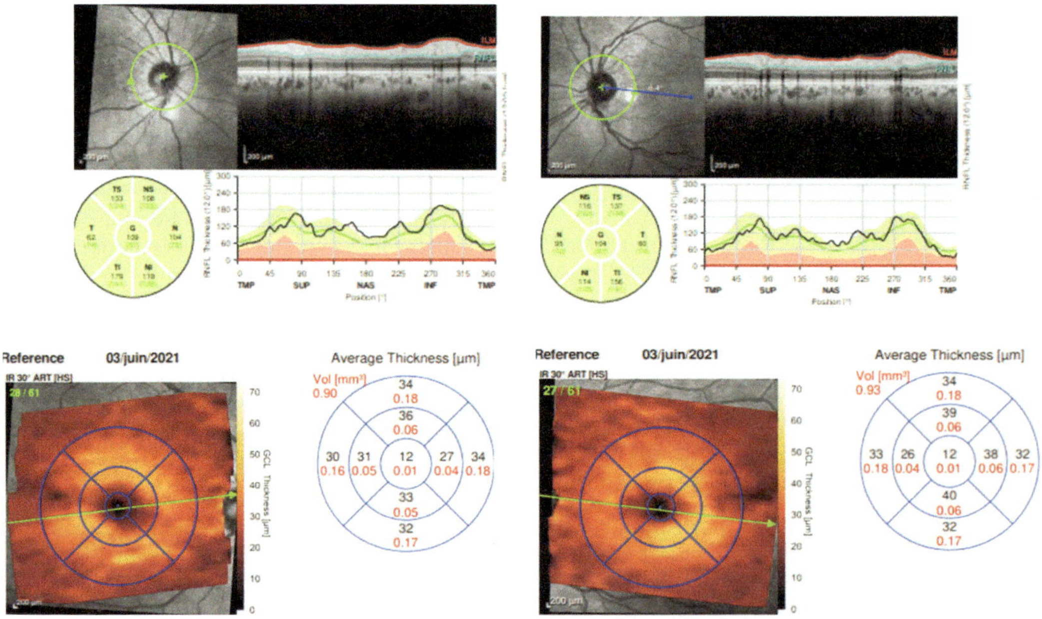
TMP
SUP
NAS
INF
TMP
Reference 03/juin/2021
Average Thickness [µm]
Vol [mm³]
0.90
34
0.18
36
0.06
30
0.16
31
0.05
12
0.01
27
0.04
34
0.18
33
0.05
32
0.17
Reference 03/juin/2021
Average Thickness [µm]
Vol [mm³]
0.93
34
0.18
39
0.06
33
0.18
26
0.04
12
0.01
38
0.06
32
0.17
40
0.06
32
0.17

C

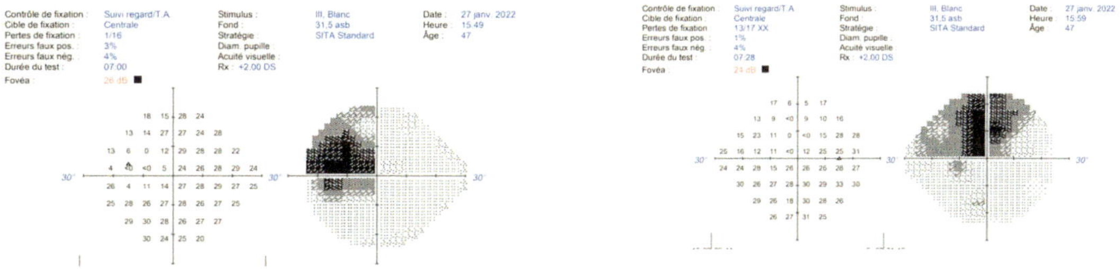

D

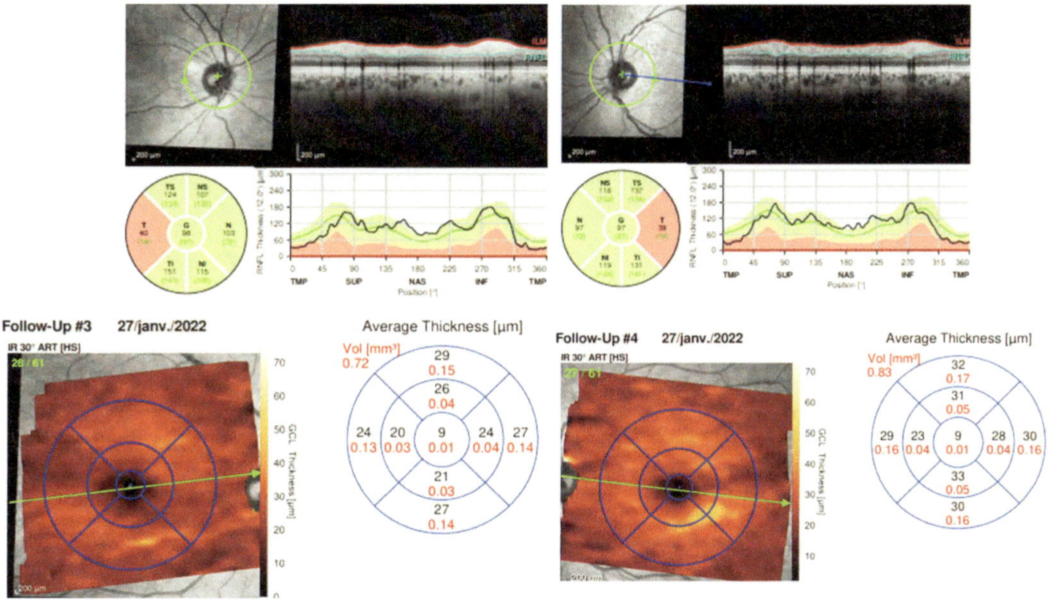
Follow-Up #3 27/janv./2022
IR 30° ART [HS]
Average Thickness [µm]
Vol [mm³]
0.72
GCL Thickness [µm]
Follow-Up #4 27/janv./2022
IR 30° ART [HS]
Average Thickness [µm]
Vol [mm³]
0.83

E

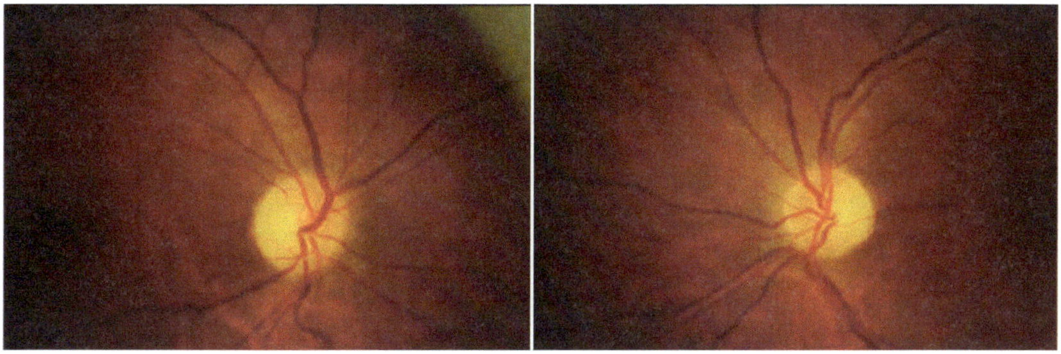

F

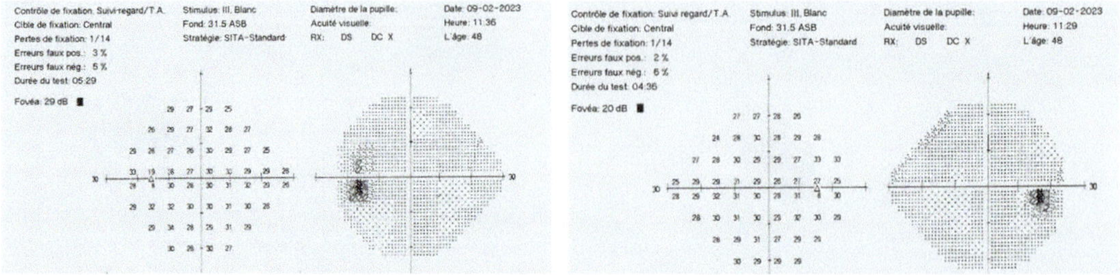

G

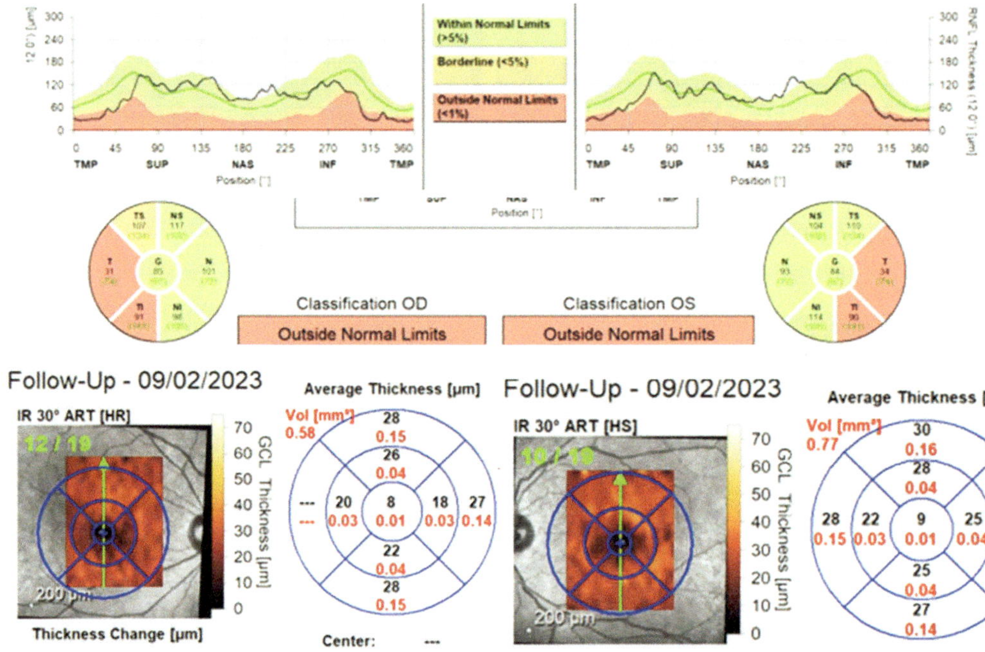

H

Figure 6.3: Spontaneous recovery in a 47-year-old male patient with m.14484T>C. In Nov 2020 he complained of bilateral rapid painless loss of vision OU. Risk factors included tobacco and alcohol exposure, no family history of LHON but ultimately diagnosed with LHON m.14484T>C variant in ND6.

A: First visit in April 2021, BCVA 20/160 OD and 20/50 OS. Bilateral optic disc pallor. **B**: Humphrey 24-2 central scotomas, **C**: normal RNFL and diffuse thinning of GCC OU. **D**: Jan 2022 progressive vision loss to BCVA HM OD and 20/125 OS. Humphrey visual field demonstrating bilateral central scotoma, **E**: temporal RNFL thinning and diffuse loss of macular GCC OU. **F**: Feb 2023, partial spontaneous recovery "normal Snellen" BCVA 20/20OU, with bilateral optic disc pallor. Low foveal threshold (20dB OD, 29 dB OS), but no scotoma on Humphrey visual field testing (**G**) despite more pronounced loss of RGC (RNFL and macula) (**H**).

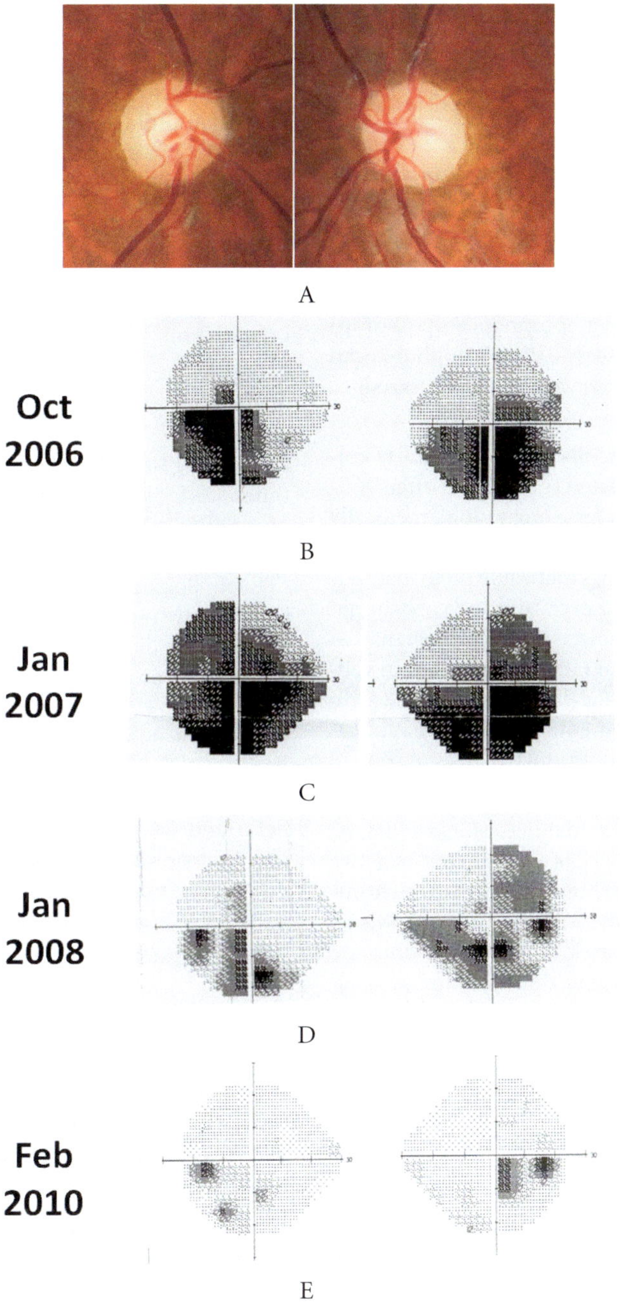

Figure 6.4: Spontaneous recovery with fenestration in a 15-year-old male patient with m.14484T>C. Initial symptoms presented in June 2006 with bilateral rapid painless loss of vision. He had no family history of LHON but was ultimately diagnosed with LHON m.14484T>C variant in ND6. BCVA OD 20/120, OS 20/400.
A: Bilateral optic disc pallor and Humphrey visual fields with bilateral cecocentral scotomas (**B**). Jan 2007, worsening of VA 20/800 OU (**C**). In Jan 2008 BCVA improvement to 20/30 OU and fenestration apparent in the scotoma on Humphrey visual field testing (**D**). Feb 2010, continued visual improvement to 20/20 OD and 20/25 OS with decrease in the size of the scotomas (**E**).

6.4. Longterm sequelae

Visual field and visual acuity are only two metrics by which vision is measured. It is important to recognize that the natural history of LHON also affects other aspects of vision, which are not usually assessed. For instance, almost all subjects have some degree of dyschromatopsia, which usually begins with a gradual loss of color sensitivity and evolves over time to range from color confusion to compete achromatopsia. The dyschromatopsia can be accompanied by photophobia, dysphotopsia and glare. In some cases, the photophobia can be treated with tinted eyewear designed to reduce glare.

Similarly, poor visual acuity does not equate to colloquial blindness. Affected subjects are often concerned that they will have no vision, medically equating to no light perception (NLP). The natural history data clearly shows that while the visual acuity is poor, it is almost never NLP and care should be taken to reassure subjects of this important distinction. Indeed, most LHON patients retain substantial peripheral visual field, allowing them to navigate their environment. Most LHON subjects are able to lead full and productive lives in spite of any limitations imposed by their reduced vision.

In addition to the ocular manifestations of LHON, subjects may also experience significant negative psychological and psychosocial effects which impact quality of life. Some features such as the visual hallucinations of Charles Bonnet syndrome are often underdiagnosed and thus not clinically addressed. Alcohol abuse is not uncommon. Subjects frequently experience anxiety, depression, and even suicidal ideation in response to their sudden vision loss, all of which needs to be appropriately addressed. Screening for potential sequelae is important for maintaining the physical and psychosocial health of subjects.

A subject affected by LHON is also susceptible to other diseases and in some cases, they can be potentiated by the presence of an LHON variant. Interactions have been reported for LHON with cardiac abnormalities, and neurological issues including myopathy (☞ Chapter 5.). One challenge with this data is that some of these interactions are based upon small case series from a few pedigrees, which may overestimate the prevalence of a common disease with a rare disease. While the link has not been formally established, screening for cardiac disease is prudent and should be considered in all carriers of LHON variants, regardless if they are affected. Harding described an overlap between multiple sclerosis and the optic neuropathy of LHON. Statistically one would expect a relatively common (MS) and relatively rare (LHON) disease to occur in the same individual by random chance alone. Clinically, however, subjects with LHON-MS may have a more aggressive course, suggesting mechanistic interaction and potentiation (14).

LHON subjects are susceptible to other age-related ocular diseases which may get masked by the presence of LHON. Cataract formation, for example, is a natural age-related phenomenon which is sometimes overlooked in subjects with LHON. Attrition of the RNFL is a normal age-related process and continues in subjects with optic atrophy from LHON. Subjects with advanced glaucoma, for instance, are more susceptible to lower even "normal" intraocular pressures (IOP) (15). A similar correlation can be found in subjects with advanced optic atrophy for any reason including LHON. Monitoring subjects with LHON for progressive RNFL loss and increased optic disc cupping can be challenging due to the floor effects in both visual fields and OCT RNFL measurements. Diagnosis plus appropriate and timely treatment of other potentially treatable ocular diseases in subjects with LHON helps to maximize visual potential and decrease the risk of further vision loss.

6.5. Challenges

LHON is a rare, complex, multisystem disease which impacts the physical and psychosocial health of subjects. Our understanding of the natural history of the disease is largely based upon small retrospective studies and case reports. The meta-analysis of m.11778G>A subjects, for example, contained data of only 695 subjects, with 3 prospective studies accounting for about 10% of the subjects included in the analysis (6). An over-reliance on retrospective data is prone to error as environmental impacts have changed over the years including rates of smoking, a strongly linked risk factor for LHON. Large scale prospective natural history studies are not possible in LHON due to the low incidence of the disease and the relatively recent availability of therapeutic interventions to treat the disease. The international consensus statement on LHON recommends treatment with idebenone, which makes further natural history studies ethically challenging.

Published data shows that LHON is a heterogeneous disease with variable penetrance and clinical manifestations (☞ Chapter 5.). The natural history of LHON varies widely, and is influenced by the underlying genetic variant, sex, environmental influences, and age of onset.

References

1. Carelli V, Carbonelli M, de Coo IF, Kawasaki A, Klopstock T, Lagreze WA, et al. International consensus statement on the clinical and therapeutic management of Leber hereditary optic neuropathy. J Neuroophthalmol. 2017;37(4):371-81.

2. Hwang TJ, Karanjia R, Moraes-Filho MN, Gale J, Tran JS, Chu ER, et al. Natural history of conversion of leber's hereditary optic neuropathy: A prospective case series. Ophthalmology. 2017;124(6):843-50.

3. Barboni P, Savini G, Valentino ML, La Morgia C, Bellusci C, De Negri AM, et al. Leber's hereditary optic neuropathy with childhood onset. Invest Ophthalmol Vis Sci. 2006;47(12):5303-9.

4. Cunha AM, Vilares-Morgado R, Moleiro AF, Falcão-Reis F, Faria O. Childhood-onset Leber hereditary optic neuropathy: Particular features. Int Med Case Rep J. 2021;14:163-9.

5. Kogachi K, Ter-Zakarian A, Asanad S, Sadun A, Karanjia R. Toxic medications in Leber's hereditary optic neuropathy. Mitochondrion. 2019;46:270-7.

6. Newman NJ, Carelli V, Taiel M, Yu-Wai-Man P. Visual outcomes in Leber hereditary optic neuropathy patients with the m.11778G>A (MTND4) mitochondrial DNA mutation. J Neuroophthalmol. 2020;40(4):547-57.

7. Oostra RJ, Bolhuis PA, Wijburg FA, Zorn-Ende G, Bleeker-Wagemakers EM. Leber's hereditary optic neuropathy: correlations between mitochondrial genotype and visual outcome. J Med Genet. 1994;31(4):280-6.

8. Yu-Wai-Man P, Newman NJ, Carelli V, La Morgia C, Biousse V, Bandello FM, et al. Natural history of patients with Leber hereditary optic neuropathy-results from the REALITY study. Eye (Lond). 2022;36(4):818-26.

9. Stephenson KAJ, McAndrew J, Kenna PF, Cassidy L. The natural history of Leber's hereditary optic neuropathy in an Irish population and assessment for prognostic biomarkers. Neuroophthalmology. 2022;46(3):159-70.

10. Carelli V, Newman NJ, Yu-Wai-Man P, Biousse V, Moster ML, Subramanian PS, et al. Indirect comparison of lenadogene nolparvovec gene therapy versus natural history in patients with Leber hereditary optic neuropathy carrying the m.11778G>A MT-ND4 mutation. Ophthalmol Ther. 2023;12(1):401-29.

11. Nettleship E, Thompson AH. A pedigree of Leber's disease. Proc R Soc Med. 1913;6(Sect Ophthalmol):8-16.

12. Catarino CB, Klopstock T. Use of idebenone for the treatment of Leber's hereditary optic neuropathy: review of the evidence. Journal of Inborn Errors of Metabolism and Screening. 2017;5:2326409817731112.

13. Carelli V, d'Adamo P, Valentino ML, La Morgia C, Ross-Cisneros FN, Caporali L, et al. Parsing the differences in affected with LHON: genetic versus environmental triggers of disease conversion. Brain. 2016;139(Pt 3):e17.

14. Pfeffer G, Burke A, Yu-Wai-Man P, Compston DA, Chinnery PF. Clinical features of MS associated with Leber hereditary optic neuropathy mtDNA mutations. Neurology. 2013;81(24):2073-81.

15. Yohannan J, Boland MV, Ramulu P. The association between intraocular pressure and visual field worsening in treated glaucoma patients. J Glaucoma. 2021;30(9):759-68.

7. Diagnostic pathway and differential diagnosis in LHON

Chiara La Morgia, Claudia Priglinger

LHON is an inherited mitochondrial optic nerve disease characterized by acute/subacute visual loss due to dysfunction and later degeneration of retinal ganglion cells (RGCs), in particular those contributing to the papillomacular bundle (PMB), leading to optic atrophy (1). Clinical diagnosis is not always straightforward due to the overlapping feature with other acute optic neuropathies. However, LHON should be suspected in all patients presenting with a clinical picture of bilateral and painless central visual loss without recovery, irrespective of age (1-3). For the differential diagnosis, some distinctive clinical features may help the clinician in the diagnostic pathway.

7.1. Symptoms and signs

7.1.1. Visual acuity loss

Individuals carrying LHON mutations are usually asymptomatic until they develop subacute visual loss with blurring of the central visual field in one eye. Vision loss in LHON presents initially as a relative central scotoma in one eye which then progresses to a large, dense centrocoecal scotoma and then to a generalized defect. Patients often complain of blurred vision or a central gray spot in the central visual field, which enlarges day by day. The vision loss is typically painless and in the majority of cases acute/subacute. Nadir is usually reached within 6 months. Involvement of the second eye occurs within weeks or months after the first eye (3). This pattern is almost pathognomonic of LHON, even though bilateral onset is also reported in inflammatory optic neuropathies, and particularly in the neuromyelitis optica spectrum disease (NMOSD) and in MOG-related disease (MOGAD) (4). Unilateral cases are rarely reported in LHON and in 25% of cases visual loss is bilateral at onset (3). The most characteristic feature is an enlarging central scotoma, and as the field defect increases in size and density, visual acuity declines to counting fingers or worse (5-7). The clinical diagnosis of LHON is established in a patient with above mentioned symptoms, clinical findings as follows and a pathogenic mtDNA variant identified by molecular genetic testing. In rare cases, LHON can also be inherited by an autosomal recessive trait (for molecular genetic testing and a.r. LHON ☞ Chapters 2. and 8., respectively).

7.1.2. Visual field defect

A central or centrocecal scotoma is characteristic at the onset of vision loss. Initially, when mild and still small, the scotoma may not be detectable on a 30-2 visual field, but it is usually always discernable on a 10-2 central visual field. Conversely, in advanced stages, when the scotoma is dense and large, the defect will not be demonstrable with a 30-2 stimulus III (floor effect), but can be evident with a stimulus V visual field. The scotoma usually enlarges over time and becomes a diffuse central visual field defect. Some patients can learn a compensatory strategy of eccentric fixation that delocalizes the scotoma. Different patterns of recovery also have been described, including reduction of the central scotoma or fenestration of the scotoma. Visual field improvement can be sometimes independent from visual acuity (8, 9).

7.1.3. Fundus exam findings: optic disc hyperemia, microangiopathy and pseudoedema

Ophthalmoscopy in the subacute stage often reveals vascular tortuosity of the central retinal vessels, swelling of the optic nerve fiber layer and a circumpapillary teleangiectatic microangiopathy (☞ Figure 7.1). However, in a minority of LHON cases the optic disc may look normal at presentation, while optic disc pallor becomes apparent within 6 weeks, initially more marked temporally due to the early axonal loss in the papillomacular bundle (PMB) (10).

Optic nerve fiber layer swelling typically starts in the temporal and inferior fiber arcades of the optic nerve head, moving then superiorly and finally nasally. Following disease conversion, the swelling spreads circumferentially to involve the remaining quadrants before atrophy becomes established within 3-9 months after onset of visual loss. In the acute stage, the optic disc swelling resembles optic

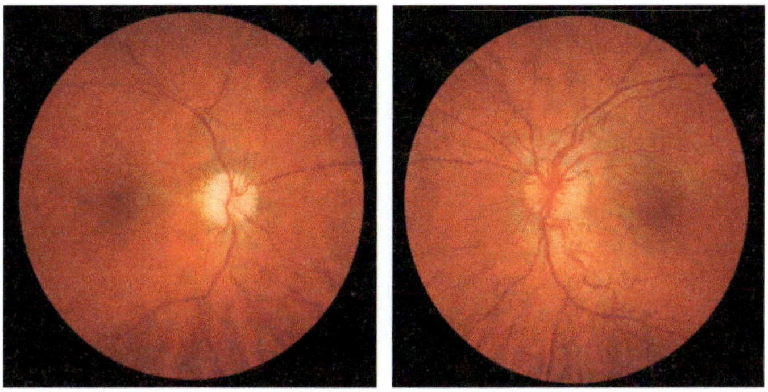

A

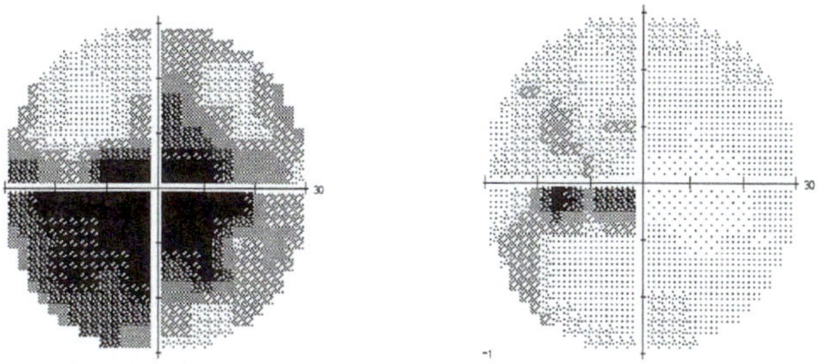

B

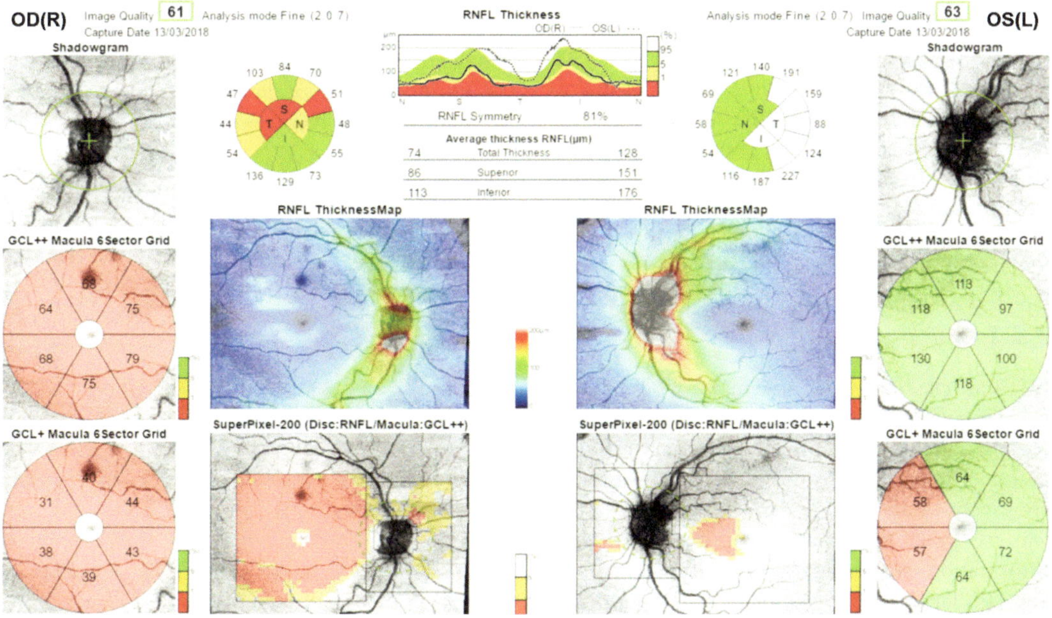

C

Figure 7.1: **A**: Fundus picture of a LHON patient in the subacute/dynamic phase, 7 months after disease onset for the RE and 2 months after disease onset for the LE; **B**: Visual fields show bilateral central scotoma more evident on the RE; **C**: Optical coherence tomography demonstrates RNFL thinning of the temporal sector associated with GCL defect for the RE and swelling of the retinal nerve fibers in the temporal-inferior sectors with an initial defect of the GCL in the papillo-macular bundle for the LE.

disc edema, but the lack of leakage from capillaries on fluorescein angiograms supports that this is a 'pseudoedema'. Several weeks after onset of symptoms, small arterioles and capillaries on the temporal side of the optic disc become attenuated, while the vasculopathy is still increasing nasally. Gradually over the next weeks the involution of the temporal microvasculature continues and temporally a small sector of retinal nerve fiber atrophy becomes more and more apparent and enlarges over time. Axonal loss slowly progresses and in the chronic stage patients develop optic disc pallor that mostly involves the temporal side of the disc. Some eyes can still show peripapillary microangiopathy at the stage of optic atrophy (5). Hyperemia and fluctuating mild swelling of the peripapillary retinal nerve fiber layers (RNFL) can also be seen in unaffected LHON mutation carriers without visual loss or progression to full disease conversion (1, 11).

7.2. Diagnostic pathway: psychophysical findings, electrophysiological testing and retinal imaging

Visual loss in LHON is a consequence of mainly macular RGC dysfunction and later of RGC loss. Assessment of color vision, pupillary light reflex and electrophysiological testing can be helpful in isolating the contribution of different RGC subpopulations to vision loss and help to differentiate LHON from other entities.

7.2.1. Background

RGCs are classified into three major types, namely midget, parasol and small bistratified RGCs, which are thought to contribute to the parvocellular, magnocellular and koniocellular pathways, respectively. Midget cells and the parvocellular pathway are thought to process high spatial frequency information and red-green perception. At difference, the large parasol cells and the fast conducting magnocellular pathway process high temporal frequency. Yellow-blue processing has been linked with bistratified RGCs and the koniocellular pathway (12, 13). In addition, in retinal topography RGCs transmitting blue-yellow vision are meant to be located perifoveally, whereas RGCs connected to foveal cones are thought to transmit red-green color vision (13-15).

LHON is thought to mainly affect midget RGCs, which have the smallest caliber. Recent extensive neurophysiological work provided evidence, that the parasol cells and the magnocellular pathway together with the bistratified cells and koniocellular pathway in LHON disease are affected as well (1). Interestingly, at difference with the regular RGCs, a small subgroup of RGCs contributing to circadian photoreception and the regulation of the pupillary light reflex (PLR), the melanopsin-expressing RGCs (mRGCs) are relatively preserved in LHON (16). The reason why this subtype is resistant to mitochondrial dysfunction is still unknown.

7.2.2. Dyschromatopsia

Vision loss from presentation in LHON is accompanied by a severe red-green dyschromatopsia. This is a key symptom when the disease starts and can easily be diagnosed by means of commercially available color vision tests. Impaired chromatic resolution along the protan and deutan axes together with compromised achromatic spatial sensitivity is compatible with a severe loss of midget GCLs and the parvocellular axons as well as of a concomitant involvement of the large parasol cells.

Deficiency in the tritan axis suggests also the involvement of the koniocellular pathway in the subacute stage (1). When vision is severely affected (>1.4 logMAR), protan color sensitivity is typically lost, while loss of blue-yellow vision appears more gradual with 30-80% color confusion in isoluminant color optotypes (17). However, this pattern of color vision disturbance is not specific to LHON and can be found also in inflammatory optic neuropathies (18).

Reports on color visions disturbance in *asymptomatic* LHON carriers are more conflicting and may be confounded by the type of test used and range from subnormal to pathologic in a subset of patients. Only slightly subnormal findings along all chromatic axes compared with normal were evidenced with the Cambridge Color Test (1), whereas tritan defects were found in 40% and deutan defects in 56% of asymptomatic carriers with the m.11778G>A mutation using the Farnsworth-Munsell 100 hue test. From these findings the authors concluded that the tritan defects observed in LHON carriers may be a marker for subclinical PMB dysfunction, whereas the deutan defects may be indicative of a selective degeneration of the small calibre fibers and RGCs transmitting the signals from the red-green cones in the central 2° of the visual field (14). With equiluminance adjustments for the red/green axis Ventura and colleagues were able to provide evidence that asymptomatic carriers required higher intensities in the green than controls, whereas the equiluminance settings for blue/yellow did not differ from controls.

This is in line with the concept that the parvocelluar component of the PMB is affected first and subclinical dysfunction in red-green vision is present in asymptomatic carriers, as well as that larger sized RGCs such as the bistratified and other S-cone opponent RGC types, which process blue/yellow vision may be spared in the subclinical stage (15). Whether subtle color deficiencies as detected with commercially available color testing techniques are of prognostic value and may help identify subjects at risk for disease conversion has not yet been elucidated.

7.2.3. Pupillary light reflex and pupillometry

Melanopsin retinal ganglion cells (mRGCs) are a small subgroup (around 1%) of intrinsically photosensitive RGCs expressing the photopigment melanopsin with a relevant role in regulating the PLR (19). These cells, which are particularly responsive to blue light (460-480 nm), are characterized by a tonic and sluggish response to light and are more concentrated around the fovea (19).

Post-mortem and pupillometric studies demonstrated a relative sparing of these cells in LHON (20, 21), as confirmed also by the maintenance of the melatonin suppression test response to light in these patients (20). The maintenance of the PLR even in the chronic stage of the disease and in the presence of a severe optic atrophy is an important and quite specific clinical finding in LHON, which can help in the differential diagnosis from inflammatory optic neuropathies. In the very acute phase of the disease and in the unilateral presentation, however, a mild relative afferent pupillary defect (RAPD), which is typical for inflammatory optic neuritis, can be seen also in LHON patients.

7.2.4. Electrophysiological findings

The function of the PMB and the macular RGCs can be assessed objectively using pattern reversal visual evoked potentials (P-VEP) and pattern electroretinogram (PERG). Reported P-VEP abnormalities in LHON are consistently severe. The utility of PERG in LHON is more controversial and there are conflicting reports in the literature regarding the timing of responses and the sequence of losses. More recently, another useful electrophysiological marker for evaluating RGC function has been proposed for LHON, i.e. the photopic negative response (PhNR) (1).

7.2.4.1. Pattern visual evoked potentials

P-VEP mainly is a measure of macular RGC function and can be used to measure axonal loss. Pattern reversal VEP (P-VEP) records the bioelectrical response of the visual cortex in response to a visual stimulus thereby assessing functional integrity from the retina to the striate cortex. Typically, VEPs are recorded using high contrast pattern checkerboard stimuli, which are reversed in contrast over time (P-VEP). The typical P-VEP waveform comprises a triphasic response with components named according to their relative polarity and peak-time. A major positive peak is seen around 100 ms (P100), with preceding and following negative peaks around 75 ms (N75) and 135 ms (N135), respectively. The amplitude is considered to arise mainly from the axonal component of the RGCs, whereas the conduction time from myelinated axons (22).

In the subacute stage of LHON P-VEP P100 is severely reduced in amplitude and delayed in all affected eyes or not recordable, a finding that may be a consequence of severe axonal dysfunction (10, 23). P-VEP changes can manifest in affected eyes before a temporal pallor is clinically visible. In the chronic stage P-VEP response remains abnormal (24).

These findings, however, are not specific of LHON, since different conditions of the optic nerve and RGCs may affect response amplitude or latency preferentially and P-VEP can be affected by anything upstream in the visual pathway. For this reason, the combined use of P-VEP and PERG together with the optical coherence (OCT) findings can be of help in localizing the site of the lesion at the level of the optic nerve (22).

7.2.4.2. Pattern electroretinogram

Central retinal function due to RGC dysfunction can be assessed using pattern ERG (P-PERG). In P-ERG the stimulus consists of a contrast-reversing checker board displayed on a monitor. The P-ERG response has two major components: the positive P50 and the larger negative N95. A large body of experimental evidence suggests that the N95 arises in the macular retinal ganglion cells, while the P50 is driven by the macular photoreceptors. A reduction of the PERG N95 combined with a preserved P50 suggests dysfunction at the level or the macular retinal ganglion cells (25).

As a consequence of RGC degeneration and axonal loss in the chronic stage of LHON the N95 component of pattern electroretinography (PERG) is markedly reduced and accordingly the P100 component of the P-VEP is abnormal to not detectable (24). For the acute stage the literature on electrophysiological findings is quite controversial. In the acute stage of LHON, degeneration of RGCs is proceeded by a primary dysfunction of these cells and this is reflected by a reduced 15' N95 component of PERG, before the optic disc pallor appears, even though this finding is not present in all patients (10, 24, 26). This is supported by the electrophysiological findings reported in a Slovenian case series in the very acute stage of LHON (disease duration 2-10 weeks) in which the N95 component was reduced in 50% of the affected eyes, whilst PERG P50 component was normal in all, in line with a macular parvocellular RGC dysfunction and preserved macular photoreceptor function. Interestingly, in all acutely affected eyes with normal PERG N95 no pallor was observed at the time of PERG, suggesting that the majority of RGCs was still viable. Conversely, in 4/7 eyes with reduced PERG N95 temporal pallor of the optic disc was visible (10). Conversely, another recent study found consistent PERG abnormalities in all patients with acute LHON, including a shortened P50 peak time and reduced N95/P50 ratio in patients with acute LHON. In agreement with the Slovenian cohort the P50 amplitude was preserved (1).

Taken together, a reduced 15' PERG N95 amplitude or N95/P50 ratio can be expected in 50-100% of LHON patients in the acute stage and especially in those with temporal optic disc pallor. However, at the same time a normal PERG in this stage does not exclude LHON. Of interest, a reduction of the 15' PERG P50-N95 amplitude values only, was observed in a cohort of unaffected LHON carriers, while P-VEP and 60' PERG were normal in all (24). This further confirms the presumable relevance of 15' PERG in as a diagnostic tool in acute LHON and suggests that there is an early RGC dysfunction in subgroups of asymptomatic LHON carriers of LHON. However, to this date, there are no published data to evaluate whether reduced 15' PERG P50-N95 amplitude values are predictive of an impending disease conversion in unaffected mutation carriers.

7.2.4.3. PhNR

The photopic negative response (PhNR) is a slow negative wave response observable on the flash-ERG immediately following the b-wave of the cone response reflecting the exclusive contribution of RGCs. Recent studies demonstrated a reduction in PhNR amplitude in both affected LHON patients and asymptomatic carriers (1, 27).

7.2.5. Retinal imaging

7.2.5.1. Optical coherence tomography

SD-OCT is broadly available and has become a useful tool in the diagnosis and in the follow-up of LHON patients. In particular, the macular ganglion cell-inner plexiform layer (mGCL-IPL) thickness map may help in detecting the earliest morphological changes in LHON and is an important aid in differential diagnosis of other optic neuropathies.

OCT of the macula

The first studies focusing on retinal structure in vivo have shown that even in the *pre-symptomatic* stage of LHON, i.e. 4-6 weeks before the onset of visual loss, thinning of the macular GCL-IPL is observed by SD-OCT in the fellow eye. In two case reports the earliest sign was a thinning of the inner ETDRS ring in the nasal sectors, where the RGC bodies that contribute to the papillomacular bundle reside (28, 29). This defect progressively extended to the outer ring of the nasal sector over a period of one month, when loss of vision occurs. At this stage, the 10-2 visual field sometimes already demonstrates a subclinical central scotoma, before the RGC loss leads to visual loss (29). Conversely, the inner nuclear layer (INL) was reported to be thicker in chronic affected LHON compared with controls or unaffected LHON carriers (2, 30).

In the *subacute stage* of LHON, macular SD-OCT scans reveal progressive thinning of the mGCL-IPL complex within a few weeks of disease onset. The greatest GCL-IPL thickness change can be detected between the presymptomatic stage and the first 3 months of the disease continuing up to six months after onset and then gradually reaching a plateau. Balducci and colleagues described a sequential pattern of GCL loss proceeding from the inner ring of the inferior sector to the outer ring of the nasal sectors, inner ring of the temporal and the superior sectors, followed by the outer ring of the temporal sectors, and finally the outer ring of the superior and inferior sectors. This centrifugal and spiral pattern reflects the distribution of contributing RGCs to the PMB (29). Thus, in the early subacute stage (0-4 months after onset of vision loss) 50% of the macular GCL-IPL is lost (1). Interestingly, INL thickness remains increased even in patients with chronic LHON (2, 29). In the *chronic stage* of LHON, OCT analysis detects complete atrophy of the GCL-IPL in all sectors.

OCT of the peripapillary RNFL (pRNFL)

In the *pre-symptomatic* stage, pRNFL thickening may be visible up to 4-6 months preceding conversion with an even sharper increase 0-2 months before disease onset (31). In the first 3 months after onset, GCL-IPL thinning usually precedes peripapillary (p)RNFL with the *temporal* sector of the optic nerve being the first presenting loss of fibers corresponding to temporal pallor at fundus examination. At this *early subacute* stage, OCT findings confirm ophthalmoscopic evidence of optic nerve fiber swelling. Peripapillary RNFL thickening is possibly secondary to axonal swelling due to an impaired axonal transport of mitochondria, with an accumulation of them within the dysfunctional RGCs, particularly involving the prelaminar unmyelinated portion of the optic nerve (32). The pattern of swelling and thinning of the optic nerve fibers follows a specific sequence with the inferotemporal sectors being the first undergoing thickening and thus the first presenting atrophy and the nasal sector the last (33). Specifically, considering the 12 sectors of the pRNFL circle, in the presymptomic stage a thickening of sector 8 is evident, coincided with an increase in the thickness of the sectors bordering the PMB (6 and 7 for the inferior sectors, 10 and 11 for the superior sectors) synchronous with the thinning of sectors 8 and then 9 (34). Thus, in the early subacute stage *global* peripapillary RNFL thickening is evident, while thinning is visible within 3 months of disease onset and more obvious in the dynamic stage (6-12 months). Furthermore, pRNFL thinning can continue even after 60 months (2). Patients with visual recovery and smaller central scotomas usually maintain a thicker average RNFL compared to patients without recovery (35).

A recent OCT study looking at structural data from *chronic* LHON patients in comparison with those affected by other phenotypically similar optic neuropathies showed that in chronic LHON besides the well-established thinning of all other ETDRS fields a relative thickening of RNFL, GCL-IPL and INL in the central ETDRS (Early Treatment Diabetic Retinopathy Study) circle is evident. This appeared to be a feature indicative of chronic LHON. A ratio between the middle ETDRS ring and the central circle thicknesses for RNFL and GCL closer to 1.5 may be indicative for LHON, whilst ratios over 2 are more suggestive for other optic neuropathies, which might be helpful for distinguishing chronic LHON from other types of optic neuropathy if molecular genetic testing is not available or negative (2).

ONH analysis

OCT studies looking at the ONH and specifically at the ON disc size in LHON demonstrated the presence of a bigger optic disc in LHON patients carrying the 14484/ND6 mutation. Interestingly, having a bigger optic disc has been demonstrated to be a positive prognostic factor in LHON. In fact, mean optic disc area was significantly larger in LHON carriers than in LHON-affected and controls. Furthermore, the LHON-affected with visual recovery had a significantly larger vertical disc diameter when compared with those without visual recovery (36).

OCT-A

A few OCT-A studies are available in LHON. Balducci and colleagues reported a reduced peripapillary vessel density in LHON patients in the early stage of the disease (29). Moreover, Borrelli and colleagues showed that choroidal thickening follows RNFL changes in the early stages of the disease (37).

7.2.6. Optic disc perfusion – laser speckle flowgraphy (LSFG)

A study by Calzetti and colleagues, using laser speckle contrast imaging (LSCI) which allows to measure optic disk blood flow, demonstrated that optic disc microvascular perfusion is increased in the early subacute stage of the disease and declined below the values of controls during the late subacute stage (P=0.024). This finding may be the consequence of vasodilation due to nitric oxide release as compensation to mitochondrial impairment typical of LHON (30).

7.3. Differential diagnosis of LHON

7.3.1. Optic neuritis (ON) and other inflammatory disorders of the optic nerve

Inflammatory optic neuropathies are the main differential diagnosis for LHON. In the acute phase, they can give rise to significant visual impairment, red-green dyschromatopsia and a centrocoecal scotoma, warranting early identification of etiology in order to start the appropriate treatment. As opposed to LHON, ON typically causes ocular pain exacerbated by eye movements and is characterized by a clear RAPD (38). About one third of optic neuritis cases are characterized by optic disc edema which is usually more prominent than the pseudoedema typical of LHON. Moreover, the classical retrobulbar optic neuritis is usually unilateral, with the exception of AQP4/MOG-related optic neuritis/papillitis which can also be bilateral at onset (39).

Typically, the classical demyelinating optic neuritis associated with multiple sclerosis (MS) quite rapidly improves spontaneously or after steroid therapy (in the first weeks), as opposed to LHON for which the spontaneous recovery rarely occurs and usually months/years after onset. Another important clue for differential diagnosis is the absence of fluorescein leakage at FAG at difference with inflammatory papillitis (40).

ON causes a retrograde degeneration of RGCs leading to pRNFL loss that can be detected by OCT approximately after 3 months from onset, whereas the typical sequence of swelling and thinning observed in LHON is not evident in inflammatory papillitis as well as the very GCL defect observed in the early subacute stage of LHON. Studies comparing the affected and non-affected eye in patients with acute ON detected thinning of the GCL-IPL within 5 weeks of onset (41). Furthermore, similar to LHON, in the acute phase of optic neuritis, the P-VEP is significantly attenuated or delayed, most likely upon a conduction block of the axonal volley (42). After the acute phase, however, amplitude often improves, but the delay most commonly persists despite of the resolution of visual acuity or field defects (43). This is in clear contrast to LHON, where P-VEP latencies remain delayed and amplitudes reduced as does visual acuity. Furthermore, in optic neuritis, it usually takes up to 6 weeks for a PERG abnormality to appear after onset of vision loss. This reflects the time taken for retrograde degeneration to occur to RGC axons, which then predominantly affects the N95 component. Thus, as the PERG N95 loss in optic neuritis typically occurs after the acute phase of vision loss, a reduced PERG N95 during acute presentation suggests other primary RGC disease such as LHON or other optic nerve pathology (44).

7.3.2. Toxic and nutritional optic neuropathies

Toxic and nutritional optic neuropathies are bilateral at onset in the majority of cases and are characterized as LHON by subacute visual loss and may be discerned by taking careful history of the patients. In the acute phase it is possible to observe swelling of the optic nerve fibers, even though it is usually less pronounced than in LHON. Visual field defect is usually a central scotoma as for LHON (45). The OCT defect is usually typically limited to the temporal sector of the optic nerve and, in this respect, is not distinguishable from LHON (46). If the toxic/nutritional insult is removed, the patient typically presents a recovery of visual function. At the electrophysiological level, a marked P-VEP amplitude reduction is a hallmark finding in toxic optic neuropathies (47).

7.3.3. Ischemic optic neuropathies

Non-arteritic anterior ischemic optic neuropathies (NAION) are typically characterized by unilateral subacute visual loss associated without eye pain and with an altitudinal defect visible at visual fields. The presence of pale optic disc edema with peripapillary hemorrhage evolving to pallor over weeks is an invariable feature of this condition. Involvement of the fellow eye occurs in 15% of cases at 5 years (48).

The arteritic variant (AION) usually has a late onset (>70 years), and is often associated with systemic symptoms such as headache, scalp tenderness, jaw claudicatio, polymyalgia rheumatica, fatigue and weight loss. Supportive feature is the presence of ESR and CRP elevation. Pale ONH swelling due to choroidal and retinal ischemia and cotton wool spots are evident at fundus examination. In those cases, the clinical work-up should include a screening for giant cell arteritis and other systemic vasculitis such as SLE, PAN and Churg-Strauss syndrome (49).

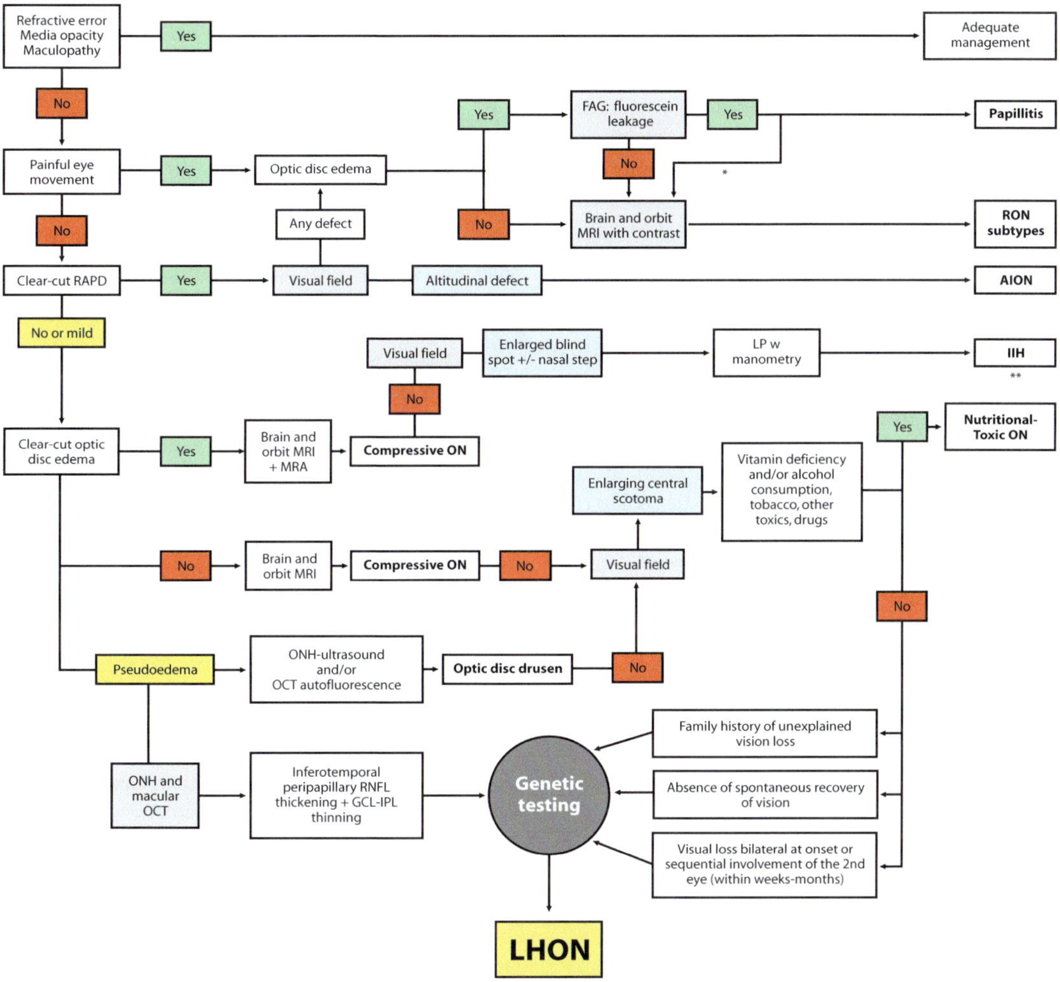

Figure 7.2: Differential diagnosis for subacute unilateral/bilateral visual loss. *In the presence of anterior papillitis (confirmed by leakage of fluorescein at FAG) brain MRI with contrast is requested to rule out the presence of inflammatory/demyelinating lesions of the brain. ** Idiopathic intracranial hypertension is usually associated with transient visual obscurations but rarely, for the fulminant presentations can be associated to severe visual acuity loss. AION: anterior ischemic optic neuropathy; IIH: idiopathic intrakranial hypertension; ONH: optic nerve head; LP: lumbar puncture; RON: retrobulbar optic neuritis.

7.3.4. Compressive optic neuropathies

A compressive optic neuropathy (CON) can occur by compressing the vascular supply and causing ischemia to the nerve or by directly compressing the axons, thereby impairing axonal transport and signal transmission. Patients with CON usually present with slow and chronic progressive vision loss in one or both eyes, but an acute worsening of vision is also possible. Commonly patients experience blurred vision and dyschromatopsia is present. Depending on the location of the compressive lesion patients suffer from additional symptoms including headache, nausea, vomiting, diplopia, red eye, or exophthalmos. The type of visual field defects largely depends on the location of the compressive lesion. Midline lesions (e.g. craniopharyngioma, pituary adenoma, meningioma) may cause peripheral visual field defects, bitemporal hemianopsia or junctional visual field loss. Orbital inflammatory disease, masses or tumors of the intraorbital portion of the optic nerve can present with optic disc edema and centrocecal scotoma, but also unilateral nerve fiber layer or altitudinal visual field defects until later on variable optic disc pallor becomes apparent. The more proximal the damage is to the eye, the quicker thinning of pRNFL and of retinal GCL layer will occur (50). Even though neuroimaging is the primary diagnostic tool to rule out CON, ancillary testing may differ among the different underlying entities. For example, tritan deficiency is a powerful tool to diagnose and monitor early dysthyroid optic neuropathy, whereas VEP was found to be not as sensitive (51, 52). In monitoring children with histologically mostly low-grade optic nerve gliomas, pRNFL measurements were shown to be more reliable to rule out progression than visual field or high contrast visual acuity testing (53).

A schematic diagnostic flow-chart is provided in Figure 7.2 for differential diagnosis in subacute unilateral/bilateral visual loss.

References

1. Majander A, Robson AG, Joao C, Holder GE, Chinnery PF, Moore AT, et al. The pattern of retinal ganglion cell dysfunction in Leber hereditary optic neuropathy. Mitochondrion. 2017;36:138-49.

2. Petrovic Pajic S, Lapajne L, Vratanar B, Fakin A, Jarc-Vidmar M, Sustar Habjan M, et al. The relative preservation of the central retinal layers in Leber hereditary optic neuropathy. J Clin Med. 2022;11(20).

3. Newman NJ, Lott MT, Wallace DC. The clinical characteristics of pedigrees of Leber's hereditary optic neuropathy with the 11778 mutation. American Journal of Ophthalmology. 1991;111(6):750-62.

4. Lana-Peixoto MA, Talim N. Neuromyelitis optica spectrum disorder and anti-MOG syndromes. Biomedicines. 2019;7(2).

5. Nikoskelainen EK, Huoponen K, Juvonen V, Lamminen T, Nummelin K, Savontaus ML. Ophthalmologic findings in Leber hereditary optic neuropathy, with special reference to mtDNA mutations. Ophthalmology. 1996;103(3):504-14.

6. Newman NJ, Yu-Wai-Man P, Carelli V, Biousse V, Moster ML, Vignal-Clermont C, et al. Intravitreal gene therapy vs. natural history in patients with Leber hereditary optic neuropathy carrying the m.11778G>A ND4 mutation: Systematic review and indirect comparison. Frontiers in Neurology. 2021;12:662838.

7. Newman NJ, Carelli V, Taiel M, Yu-Wai-Man P. Visual outcomes in Leber hereditary optic neuropathy patients with the m.11778G>A (MTND4) mitochondrial DNA mutation. J Neuroophthalmol. 2020;40(4):547-57.

8. Newman NJ, Biousse V, Newman SA, Bhatti MT, Hamilton SR, Farris BK, et al. Progression of visual field defects in leber hereditary optic neuropathy: experience of the LHON treatment trial. American Journal of Ophthalmology. 2006;141(6):1061-7.

9. Ran R, Yang S, He H, Ma S, Chen Z, Li B. A retrospective analysis of characteristics of visual field damage in patients with Leber's hereditary optic neuropathy. Springer plus. 2016;5(1):843.

10. Jarc-Vidmar M, Tajnik M, Brecelj J, Fakin A, Sustar M, Naji M, et al. Clinical and electrophysiology findings in Slovene patients with Leber hereditary optic neuropathy. Doc Ophthalmol. 2015;130(3):179-87.

11. Nikoskelainen E, Hoyt WF, Nummelin K. Ophthalmoscopic findings in Leber's hereditary optic neuropathy. I. Fundus findings in asymptomatic family members. Archives of Ophthalmology (Chicago, Ill : 1960). 1982;100(10):1597-602.

12. Wassle H, Boycott BB. Functional architecture of the mammalian retina. Physiol Rev. 1991;71(2):447-80.

13. Grigsby SS, Vingrys AJ, Benes SC, King-Smith PE. Correlation of chromatic, spatial, and temporal sensitivity in optic nerve disease. Invest Ophthalmol Vis Sci. 1991;32(13):3252-62.

14. Sadun AA, Salomao SR, Berezovsky A, Sadun F, Denegri AM, Quiros PA, et al. Subclinical carriers and conversions in Leber hereditary optic neuropathy: a pro-

spective psychophysical study. Transactions of the American Ophthalmological Society. 2006;104:51-61.

15. Ventura DF, Quiros P, Carelli V, Salomao SR, Gualtieri M, Oliveira AG, et al. Chromatic and luminance contrast sensitivities in asymptomatic carriers from a large Brazilian pedigree of 11778 Leber hereditary optic neuropathy. Invest Ophthalmol Vis Sci. 2005;46(12): 4809-14.

16. La Morgia C, Ross-Cisneros FN, Hannibal J, Montagna P, Sadun AA, Carelli V. Melanopsin-expressing retinal ganglion cells: implications for human diseases. Vision Res. 2011;51(2):296-302.

17. Rudolph G, Dimitriadis K, Buchner B, Heck S, Al-Tamami J, Seidensticker F, et al. Effects of idebenone on color vision in patients with leber hereditary optic neuropathy. Journal of Neuro-Ophthalmology. 2013;33(1): 30-6.

18. Ventura DF, Gualtieri M, Oliveira AG, Costa MF, Quiros P, Sadun F, et al. Male prevalence of acquired color vision defects in asymptomatic carriers of Leber's hereditary optic neuropathy. Invest Ophthalmol Vis Sci. 2007;48(5):2362-70.

19. Hattar S, Liao HW, Takao M, Berson DM, Yau KW. Melanopsin-containing retinal ganglion cells: architecture, projections, and intrinsic photosensitivity. Science (New York, NY). 2002;295(5557):1065-70.

20. La Morgia C, Ross-Cisneros FN, Sadun AA, Hannibal J, Munarini A, Mantovani V, et al. Melanopsin retinal ganglion cells are resistant to neurodegeneration in mitochondrial optic neuropathies. Brain. 2010;133(Pt 8):2426-38.

21. Moura AL, Nagy BV, La Morgia C, Barboni P, Oliveira AG, Salomao SR, et al. The pupil light reflex in Leber's hereditary optic neuropathy: evidence for preservation of melanopsin-expressing retinal ganglion cells. Invest Ophthalmol Vis Sci. 2013;54(7):4471-7.

22. Marmoy OR, Viswanathan S. Clinical electrophysiology of the optic nerve and retinal ganglion cells. Eye (Lond). 2021;35(9):2386-405.

23. Mashima Y, Imamura Y, Oguchi Y. Dissociation of damage to spatial and luminance channels in early Leber's hereditary optic neuropathy manifested by the visual evoked potential. Eye (Lond). 1997;11(Pt 5):707-12.

24. Ziccardi L, Sadun F, De Negri AM, Barboni P, Savini G, Borrelli E, et al. Retinal function and neural conduction along the visual pathways in affected and unaffected carriers with Leber's hereditary optic neuropathy. Invest Ophthalmol Vis Sci. 2013;54(10):6893-901.

25. Holder GE. Pattern electroretinography (PERG) and an integrated approach to visual pathway diagnosis. Prog Retin Eye Res. 2001;20(4):531-61.

26. Riordan-Eva P, Sanders MD, Govan GG, Sweeney MG, Da Costa J, Harding AE. The clinical features of Leber's hereditary optic neuropathy defined by the presence of a pathogenic mitochondrial DNA mutation. Brain. 1995;118 (Pt 2):319-37.

27. Karanjia R, Berezovsky A, Sacai PY, Cavascan NN, Liu HY, Nazarali S, et al. The photopic negative response: An objective measure of retinal ganglion cell function in patients with Leber's hereditary optic neuropathy. Invest Ophthalmol Vis Sci. 2017;58(6):BIO300-BIO6.

28. Mizoguchi A, Hashimoto Y, Shinmei Y, Nozaki M, Ishijima K, Tagawa Y, et al. Macular thickness changes in a patient with Leber's hereditary optic neuropathy. BMC Ophthalmol. 2015;15:27.

29. Balducci N, Savini G, Cascavilla ML, La Morgia C, Triolo G, Giglio R, et al. Macular nerve fibre and ganglion cell layer changes in acute Leber's hereditary optic neuropathy. Br J Ophthalmol. 2016;100(9):1232-7.

30. Calzetti G, La Morgia C, Cattaneo M, Carta A, Bosello F, Amore G, et al. Longitudinal study of optic disk perfusion and retinal structure in Leber's hereditary optic neuropathy. Invest Ophthalmol Vis Sci. 2022;63(1):43.

31. Hwang TJ, Karanjia R, Moraes-Filho MN, Gale J, Tran JS, Chu ER, et al. Natural history of conversion of Leber's hereditary optic neuropathy: A prospective case series. Ophthalmology. 2017;124(6):843-50.

32. Carelli V, Ross-Cisneros FN, Sadun AA. Mitochondrial dysfunction as a cause of optic neuropathies. Prog Retin Eye Res. 2004;23(1):53-89.

33. Barboni P, Carbonelli M, Savini G, Ramos Cdo V, Carta A, Berezovsky A, et al. Natural history of Leber's hereditary optic neuropathy: longitudinal analysis of the retinal nerve fiber layer by optical coherence tomography. Ophthalmology. 2010;117(3):623-7.

34. Carbonelli M, La Morgia C, Romagnoli M, Amore G, D'Agati P, Valentino ML, et al. Capturing the pattern of transition from carrier to affected in Leber hereditary optic neuropathy. American Journal of Ophthalmology. 2022;241:71-9.

35. Barboni P, Savini G, Valentino ML, Montagna P, Cortelli P, De Negri AM, et al. Retinal nerve fiber layer evaluation by optical coherence tomography in Leber's hereditary optic neuropathy. Ophthalmology. 2005; 112(1):120-6.

36. Ramos Cdo V, Bellusci C, Savini G, Carbonelli M, Berezovsky A, Tamaki C, et al. Association of optic disc size with development and prognosis of Leber's hereditary optic neuropathy. Invest Ophthalmol Vis Sci. 2009; 50(4):1666-74.

37. Borrelli E, Triolo G, Cascavilla ML, La Morgia C, Rizzo G, Savini G, et al. Changes in Choroidal Thickness

follow the RNFL Changes in Leber's Hereditary Optic Neuropathy. Sci Rep. 2016;6:37332.

38. Biousse V, Newman NJ. Diagnosis and clinical features of common optic neuropathies. Lancet Neurol. 2016;15(13):1355-67.

39. Rempe T, Tarhan B, Rodriguez E, Viswanathan VT, Gyang TV, Carlson A, et al. Anti-MOG associated disorder-Clinical and radiological characteristics compared to AQP4-IgG+ NMOSD-A single-center experience. Mult Scler Relat Disord. 2021;48:102718.

40. Bennett JL, Costello F, Chen JJ, Petzold A, Biousse V, Newman NJ, et al. Optic neuritis and autoimmune optic neuropathies: advances in diagnosis and treatment. Lancet Neurol. 2023;22(1):89-100.

41. Britze J, Pihl-Jensen G, Frederiksen JL. Retinal ganglion cell analysis in multiple sclerosis and optic neuritis: a systematic review and meta-analysis. Journal of Neurology. 2017;264(9):1837-53.

42. Frederiksen JL, Petrera J. Serial visual evoked potentials in 90 untreated patients with acute optic neuritis. Surv Ophthalmol. 1999;44 Suppl 1:S54-62.

43. Halliday AM, McDonald WI, Mushin J. Visual evoked response in diagnosis of multiple sclerosis. Br Med J. 1973;4(5893):661-4.

44. Holder GE. The pattern electroretinogram in anterior visual pathway dysfunction and its relationship to the pattern visual evoked potential: a personal clinical review of 743 eyes. Eye (Lond). 1997;11 (Pt 6):924-34.

45. Margolin E, Blair K, Shemesh A. Toxic and nutritional optic neuropathy. StatPearls. Treasure Island (FL) 2022.

46. Buelens T, Fils JF, Willermain F. Posterior segment spectral domain oct in the differential diagnosis of bilateral temporal optic neuropathy and its correlation with visual acuity. Int Ophthalmol. 2022;42(12):3877-89.

47. Grzybowski A, Zulsdorff M, Wilhelm H, Tonagel F. Toxic optic neuropathies: an updated review. Acta Ophthalmol. 2015;93(5):402-10.

48. Kerr NM, Chew SS, Danesh-Meyer HV. Non-arteritic anterior ischaemic optic neuropathy: a review and update. J Clin Neurosci. 2009;16(8):994-1000.

49. Bajpai V, Madan S, Beri S. Arteritic anterior ischaemic optic neuropathy: An update. Eur J Ophthalmol. 2021;31(6):2818-27.

50. Rodriguez-Beato FY, De Jesus O. Compressive optic neuropathy. StatPearls. Treasure Island (FL)2022.

51. Garip Kubler A, Halfter K, Reznicek L, Klingenstein A, Priglinger S, Rudolph G, et al. Evaluation of visual evoked potentials in dysthyroid optic neuropathy. Orbit. 2022:1-6.

52. Garip-Kuebler A, Halfter K, Reznicek L, Klingenstein A, Priglinger S, Hintschich CR. Subclinical dysthyroid optic neuropathy: tritan deficiency as an early sign of dysthyroid optic neuropathy. Br J Ophthalmol. 2021; 105(7):1019-23.

53. Avery RA, Liu GT, Fisher MJ, Quinn GE, Belasco JB, Phillips PC, et al. Retinal nerve fiber layer thickness in children with optic pathway gliomas. American Journal of Ophthalmology. 2011;151(3):542-9 e2.

8. Special topic: autosomal recessive LHON (arLHON)

Sarah Louise Stenton, Holger Prokisch

Leber's Hereditary Optic Neuropathy (LHON) is the most common disease associated with pathogenic variants in the mitochondrial DNA (mtDNA) and has been a textbook example for maternal inheritance. Recently, however, nuclear autosomal recessive causes of LHON (arLHON) have been identified that are reported to be near-indistinguishable from disease caused by variants in the mtDNA (mtLHON).

In brief, LHON is caused by loss of retinal ganglion cells, a collection of cells that are highly vulnerable to defective mitochondrial metabolism and presents with subacute, painless, simultaneous, or sequential loss of visual acuity and in the most cases is irreversible. To date, variants in two nuclear genes have been reported in patients presenting with LHON and demonstrating acute phase pathognomic features of the disease: non-hemorrhagic papillary pseudoedema, or papillary pseudoedema with peripapillary telangiectasia.

The three mtDNA encoded genes in which pathogenic variants account for the majority of maternally inherited disease (*MT-ND1*, *MT-ND4*, and *MT-ND6*) each encode a mitochondrial complex I (CI) subunit. Alike to these genes, the reported nuclear genes also play a role in mitochondrial CI function. The first is a chaperone protein required for CI maintenance (*DNAJC30*) (1-4) and the second is a central subunit of CI (*NDUFS2*) (5).

The nuclear and mtDNA encoded genes in which variants are associated with LHON are summarized in Figure 8.1.

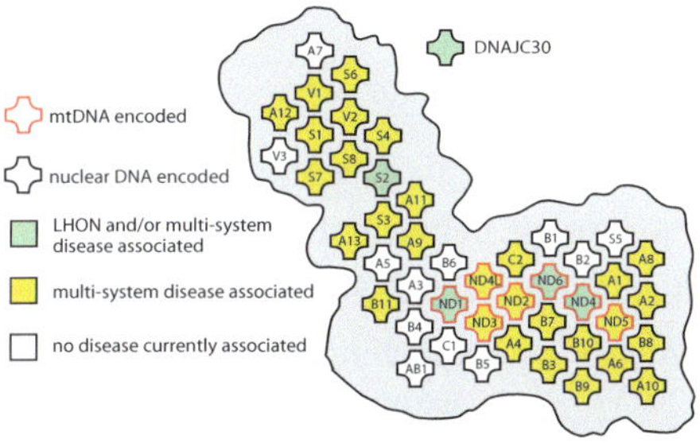

Figure 8.1: Schematic of disease associated genes involved in mitochondrial complex I function.

8.1. *DNAJC30*-associated LHON

By far, the most frequently reported cause of autosomal recessive LHON (arLHON) is biallelic variants in *DNAJC30* (MIM:619382). *DNAJC30* is a single exon gene on chromosome 7 encoding a protein proposed to be involved in mitochondrial CI maintenance and to interact with mitochondrial complex V to promote ATP synthesis (1, 6).

DNAJC30 was first reported in association with LHON in a large European cohort of unsolved, sporadic, LHON cases that had remained genetically undiagnosed following routine mtDNA or exome sequencing. In the study by Stenton et al., more than 30 cases carrying deleterious biallelic variants in *DNAJC30* were identified (1). Since this initial report, a total of almost 90 *DNAJC30*-associated LHON cases have been reported (1-4). *DNAJC30* is therefore an important gene to screen in parallel with, or sequential to, mtDNA sequencing in sporadic clinically suspected LHON.

8.1.1. Genetics

The most prevalent disease-associated variant in *DNAJC30* is Tyr51Cys. This variant is found in homozygosity in over 90% of currently reported *DNAJC30*-associated LHON cases and in a compound heterozygous state with a second deleterious variant in a further 3%. The variant is reported in patients of European decent and has a higher allele frequency in European populations compared to global frequencies (0.2% versus 0.01% in the presumably healthy gnomAD v3 population, https://gnomad.broadinstitute.org/), indicating a founder status (1-3).

In the study by Stenton et al., the Tyr51Cys missense variant was found to lead to protein instability, demonstrated by loss of the encoded protein (1). In addition to the Tyr51Cys variant, five other deleterious variants have been described. All variants are located in a highly conserved functional domain of the DNAJC30 protein, the J domain, with the exception of one nonsense variant (Glu204*) that is located upstream of the transmembrane domain of the protein.

Reported biallelic *DNAJC30* variants	Variant carriers with isolated LHON (n)	Variant carriers with LHON and LS (n)	Variant carriers with isolated LS (n)	Variant carriers remaining asymptomatic(n)
Tyr51Cys (hom)	86 (77 M, 9 F)	2 (2 M)	2 (2 F)	7 (3 M, 4 F)
Pro78Ser (hom)	2 (2 M)	–	–	–
Leu101Gln (hom)	2 (2 M)	–	–	–
Tyr51Cys + Glu204* (comp het)	3 (3 M)	–	–	–
His77del (hom)	2 (2 M)	–	–	–
Tyr51Cys + Ser44ValfsTer8 (comp het)	–	–	2 (1 M, 1 F)	–
Total	95 (86 M, 9 F)	2 (2 M)	4 (1 M, 3 F)	7 (3 M, 4 F)

Table 8.1: Reported disease-associated variants in DNAJC30.
All variant annotations apply to the ENST00000395176.3 transcript. hom: homozygous; comp het: compound heterozygous; M: male; F: female; n: number.

Table 8.1 depicts the number of variant carriers reported per biallelic disease-associated *DNAJC30* variant pair to date (1-4). We expect that this is not an exhaustive list and that further deleterious variants will be discovered in the future as *DNAJC30* is sequenced more routinely in clinical practice.

In addition to LHON, it is important to note that *DNAJC30* variants can cause Leigh syndrome (LS), a neurodegenerative mitochondrial disease characterized by bilateral symmetrical lesions within the basal ganglia and brainstem, with or without optic involvement. As depicted in Table 8.1, two unrelated LHON patients are reported with clinical features spanning both LHON and LS (carrying the homozygous Tyr51Cys *DNAJC30* variant) and four patients have been reported with LS in the absence of clinical features of LHON (two unrelated patients with homozygous Tyr51Cys variants and two siblings with compound heterozygous Tyr51Cys and Ser44ValfsTer8 variants). A clinical spectrum spanning LHON to LS and LHON/LS overlap syndromes has also been documented for mtDNA encoded causes of LHON in a small number of case reports (7, 8). For *DNAJC30*-associated LS, digenic inheritance is emerging as a potential explanation of the more severe clinical presentation, as five of the six *DNAJC30* variant carriers with LS carry an additional rare predicted deleterious variant in a mitochondrial CI subunit encoding gene (2, 4).

DNAJC30-associated LHON demonstrates incomplete penetrance (☞ Table 8.1) (1, 2). This has been explored for the frequent Tyr51Cys variant and penetrance is estimated at ~95% in males and ~60% in females carrying the variant in homozygosity (2). These penetrance values were calculated based only on families with affected members and so the penetrance is likely lower in the general population. Incomplete penetrance results in asymptomatic carriage in a small number of unaffected family members. The variant is also present in homozygosity in three presumably healthy individuals from the large population database gnomAD (v3, https://gnomad.broadinstitute.org/). The imbalance in penetrance between males and females leads to a significant male predominance of disease and an affected male to female ratio of approximately 9:1.

8.1.2. Clinical phenotype

Clinical investigation of patients with *DNAJC30*-associated LHON has confirmed presence of the subacute phase pathognomic features of LHON and has demonstrated some subtle differences in comparison to LHON caused by variants in the mtDNA:

- a younger age of disease onset
- a more frequent bilateral onset
- a higher visual acuity at nadir
- a higher rate of clinically relevant recovery (CRR) of visual acuity.

The corresponding clinical parameters are depicted in Table 8.2 and are based upon two large

Clinical parameter	Stenton et al., 2022	Kieniger et al., 2022
Reported *DNAJC30*-associated LHON cases	56	35
Male	52/56 (93%)	30/35 (86%)
Onset (age)	Median 19 years (range 9-44 years)	Median 19 years (range 10-45)
Bilateral involvement	56/56 (100%)	28/28 (100%)
Bilateral onset	24/48 (50%)	8/20 (40%)
Visual acuity at nadir	29/89 (33%) off chart; 56/89 (63%) 1.0-1.68 logMAR; 4/89 (4%) <1.0 logMAR	Median 1.3 logMAR (range 1.9-0.7)
Clinically relevant recovery of visual acuity	34/46 (74%) in total; 23/30 (77%) idebenone treated, 11/16 (69%) spontaneous	9/20 (45%) in total; all spontaneous

Table 8.2: Clinical parameters of *DNAJC30* variant carriers in two large European cohort studies. For each clinical parameter, the denominator represents the number of cases for which the data were available in the respective study. In both studies, clinically relevant recovery of visual acuity was defined as improvement ≥0.2 logMAR or change from 'off-chart' (logMAR >1.68) to 'on-chart'.

European cohort studies spanning more than 90 *DNAJC30*-associated LHON cases (2, 3).

The median age of onset in arLHON is 19 years compared to 27 years in mtLHON (2). Bilateral onset is reported in 40-50% of affected individuals compared to 25% in mtLHON (3). The course of disease in arLHON is reported to be less severe than for mtLHON, in terms of visual acuity at nadir and CRR of visual acuity. Stenton et al., report 33% to be 'off-chart', 63% to be 1.0-1.68 logMAR, and 4% to be <1.0 logMAR in arLHON at nadir compared to 50% 'off-chart', 44% 1.0-1.68 logMAR, and 6% <1.0 logMAR at nadir in a large study of mtLHON patients by Catarino et al. (9). The rate of CRR in arLHON is reported at 77% in idebenone treated and 69% in untreated (spontaneous recovery) compared to 43% and 30% in mtLHON (2). A comparison between these clinical parameters in arLHON and mtLHON is depicted in Figure 8.2.

High rates of CRR of visual acuity in *DNAJC30*-associated LHON may reflect an overall less severe natural history of the disease. Indeed, all patients experiencing CRR of visual acuity reported in the study by Kieniger et al., recovered spontaneously (untreated). In the study by Stenton et al., there was evidence supporting the use of idebenone therapy for *DNAJC30*-associated LHON, as patients receiving idebenone therapy were reported to have a positive response demonstrated by a marginally higher rate of recovery, as reported above. However, no absolute difference in the magnitude of visual acuity improvement between the idebenone-treated and spontaneous recoverees was found. These subtle trends may gain clarity as the number of identified patients increases in the future.

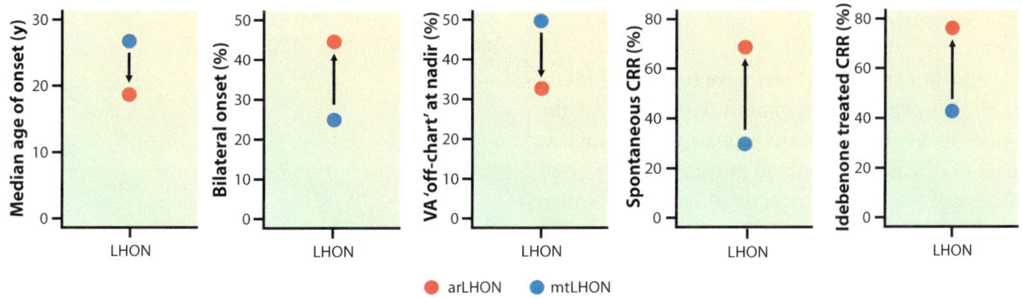

Figure 8.2: Comparison of clinical parameters in arLHON and mtLHON.
y: years; VA: visual acuity; CRR: clinically relevant recovery of visual acuity.

8.2. *NDUFS2*-associated LHON

NDUFS2 was the first nuclear gene to be linked to a non-syndromic LHON-like phenotype, however, having only been described in a single family, it remains a rare cause of autosomal recessive LHON (arLHON). Deleterious biallelic variants in *NDUFS2* are more frequently reported in cases with severe mitochondrial CI deficiency and a clinical phenotype of Leigh syndrome (LS) with optic involvement (MIM: 618228).

NDUFS2 is a 15 exon gene on chromosome 1 and, alike to MT-ND1, MT-ND4, and MT-ND6, encodes a mitochondrial CI subunit.

8.2.1. Genetics

In a study by Gerber et al., compound heterozygous missense variants (Tyr53Cys and Tyr308Cys) in *NDUFS2* were detected in three affected siblings. Functional data demonstrated normal CI activity and supported reduced NDUFS2 protein abundance resulting in a mild destabilization of mitochondrial CI. The authors suggest that the combination of a severe (Tyr53Cys) and a mild hypomorphic (Tyr308Cys) *NDUFS2* variant may explain the milder non-syndromic LHON-like phenotype in this family.

8.2.2. Clinical phenotype

The siblings experienced subacute, painless, simultaneous (2/3 siblings) or sequential (1/3 siblings) loss of visual acuity between the ages of 6 and 22 years. Two of the three siblings experienced partial spontaneous recovery of visual acuity and one experienced worsening.

Summary

The report of autosomal recessive forms of LHON (arLHON) expands the genetic landscape of the disease and promotes investigation of nuclear causes of disease in unsolved families. As reported disease genes to date, across the nuclear and mito chondrial DNA, share a pathophysiological mechanism related to mitochondrial CI deficiency, deleterious variants in genes involved in this mechanism are strong candidates for further investigation.

References

1. Stenton SL, Sheremet NL, Catarino CB, Andreeva NA, Assouline Z, Barboni P, et al. Impaired complex I repair causes recessive Leber's hereditary optic neuropathy. The Journal of Clinical Investigation. 2021;131(6).

2. Stenton SL, Tesarova M, Sheremet NL, Catarino CB, Carelli V, Ciara E, et al. DNAJC30 defect: a frequent cause of recessive Leber hereditary optic neuropathy and Leigh syndrome. Brain. 2022;145(5):1624-1631.

3. Kieninger S, Xiao T, Weisschuh N, Kohl S, Rüther K, Kroisel PM, et al. DNAJC30 disease-causing gene variants in a large Central European cohort of patients with suspected Leber's hereditary optic neuropathy and optic atrophy. Journal of Medical Genetics. 2022

4. Zawadzka M, Krygier M, Pawlowicz M, Vernet Machado M, Wilke MV, Rutkowska K, Gueguen N, et al. Expanding the phenotype of DNAJC30-associated Leigh syndrome. Clinical Genetics. 2022;102(5):438-443.

5. Gerber S, Ding MG, Gérard X, Zwicker K, Zanlonghi X, Rio M, et al. Compound heterozygosity for severe and hypomorphic NDUFS2 mutations cause non-syndromic LHON-like optic neuropathy. Journal of Medical Genetics. 2017;54(5):346-356.

6. Tebbenkamp AT, Varela L, Choi J, Paredes MI, Giani AM, Song JE, et al. The 7q11. 23 protein DNAJC30 interacts with ATP synthase and links mitochondria to brain development. Cell. 2018;175(4);1088-1104.

7. Fruhman G, Landsverk ML, Lotze TE, Hunter JV, Wangler MF, Adesina AM, et al. Atypical presentation of Leigh syndrome associated with a Leber hereditary optic neuropathy primary mitochondrial DNA mutation. Molecular Genetics and Metabolism. 2011;103 (2):153-160.

8. Miyaue N, Yamanishi Y, Tada S, Ando R, Yabe H, Nagai M, et al. Repetitive brainstem lesions in mitochondrial DNA 11778G> A mutation of Leber hereditary optic neuropathy. Eneurologicalsci. 2019;14:74.

9. Catarino CB, von Livonius B, Priglinger C, Banik R, Matloob S, Tamhankar MA, et al. Real-world clinical experience with idebenone in the treatment of Leber hereditary optic neuropathy. Journal of Neuro-Ophthalmology. 2020;40(4):558.

9. Treatment rationale and approaches

Valerio Carelli, Patrick Yu-Wai-Man

Leber's hereditary optic neuropathy (LHON) is amongst the most common mitochondrial diseases (1, 2), being the first to be associated with mitochondrial DNA (mtDNA) missense point mutations (3) and also the first for which a treatment has been approved by the European Medicines Agency (EMA), namely the quinone analogue idebenone (4). Furthermore, as there are currently multiple ongoing gene therapy trials (4-7), LHON truly represents a translational paradigm for other optic neuropathies and, more widely, for other mitochondrial disorders (8, 9).

LHON is a fairly well-characterized disease from a genetic and clinical perspective, with defined stages to its natural history that has been endorsed by an international group of experts (8-10). Furthermore, LHON presents the advantage of benefiting from relatively sophisticated tools to measure and monitor disease evolution, providing multiple endpoints for assessing therapeutic efficacy (11-13). On the downside, LHON has peculiar clinical features including variability in the timing of disease onset and progression, and unpredictable risk factors for identifying who in the maternal lineage carrying the homoplasmic mtDNA pathogenic variant will eventually experience visual loss (8, 9). Here we delineate how disease stages may relate to therapeutic approaches and how timing of intervention may be relevant for therapeutic success. These elements might vary according to the therapeutic strategy and the disease mechanisms being targeted.

9.1. Natural history and disease staging

LHON has been defined by an international consensus statement to present four distinct disease stages (10), for which therapeutic intervention may have different rationale and expectations of success (☞ Figure 9.1). The *first* stage is the so-called "*preclinical stage*" defining the status of an "*unaffected mutation carrier*", where individuals have normal vision, but may present some subclinical signs of disease activity, as assessed by fundus examination, optical coherence tomography (OCT), and other ancillary tests (8, 9). These subclinical abnormalities, which were originally well described by Nikoskelainen et al. (14), and subsequently better quantified using OCT assessment (15), can fluctuate (16) remaining stable or resolving altogether, but in a subset of individuals, these abnormalities may become more evident and eventually convert to the "*subacute stage*" of disease (11, 17). This *second* stage of LHON lasts approximately from the onset of vision loss until about six months of disease progression (10). Visual acuity rapidly deteriorates with an expanding dense central scotoma that can remain limited or enlarge to a more generalized visual field defect (8, 9). The subacute stage is characterized by the contrasting OCT measurements depending on location when comparing the macular ganglion cell complex (GCC) with the peripapillary retinal nerve fiber layer (RNFL). The macular GCC rapidly undergoes atrophy predating the onset of visual loss (18), whereas the peripapillary RNFL is initially thickened, and then the reduction in thickness follows a specific pattern involving first the inferotemporal quadrant, then the superior and nasal quadrants, with the latter sector being usually the best preserved (11). While visual loss rapidly reaches the nadir within the subacute stage, the following *third* stage, from approximately six to twelve months, is characterized by usually stable, markedly reduced visual acuity, whereas RNFL thickness might still be decreasing, and for this reason is referred to as the "*dynamic stage*" (10). The final *fourth* stage that extends beyond the twelve months since disease onset is defined as the "*chronic stage*" (10), as visual loss has stabilized with pronounced macular GCC and RNFL thinning (18, 19). During the chronic stage, a subset of LHON patients may experience unilateral or bilateral spontaneous improvement of visual function, with variable timing and influenced by the causative mtDNA mutation. A typical pattern is the appearance of "*fenestrations*" within the central scotoma, which expand and coalesce, and if this happens close to fixation, a significant improvement in visual acuity is also observed (8, 9). If the improvement mostly involves the peripheral visual field, the extent of the scotoma will shrink, but without substantial improvement in central visual acuity. Of course, the best visual outcome is reached with a combination of both patterns of visual field improvement (8, 9).

9.2. Treatment rationale and therapeutic approaches

Depending on the stage at which intervention is initiated (i.e. "*preclinical, subacute, dynamic or chronic*"), in theory, different final outcomes could be predicted. Ideally, an effective therapy at the preclinical stage would preserve vision for all unaffected individuals carrying a LHON-causing mtDNA risk variant.

Despite the significant difficulties in designing a clinical trial aimed at the preclinical stage, this would be the ideal timeframe for a gene therapy approach aimed at editing the pathogenic mtDNA variant (20, 21) in retinal ganglion cells (RGCs), the primary cellular target of LHON in the retina (8, 9). Alternatively, a drug that efficiently rebalances the pathogenic mechanisms that precipitate RGC loss would be an obvious candidate. Based on current understanding of the pathogenic mechanisms that lead to RGC loss, rational treatment options would involve reversing complex I dysfunction, suppressing reactive oxygen species (ROS) production and pathological mitophagy, and promoting compensatory mitobiogenesis and axonal transport. These approaches could all help block irreversible apoptotic cell death to avoid disease conversion (22, 23). Although several possible molecules could potentially be tested in the preclinical stage, idebenone remains to date the only EMA-approved drug for individuals already affected with LHON (4).

Once visual loss is in progress, again on a purely theoretical ground, it might be possible to abort the disease during the early subacute stage, reverting the pathological mechanism(s), or limiting cell loss during the late subacute or dynamic stage, thus preserving as much RGCs and their axons as possible, which even if not functional could eventually recover function in later stages. A postulated mechanism for either spontaneous or therapy-promoted recovery of visual function is the repair of partial myelin damage, either in terms of segmental demyelination or reduced thickness of the covering myelin sheet along axons (24). The result would be the regained capability of firing and conducting action potentials in a considerable number of surviving axons, thus re-establishing an incremental number of functional axons, which would translate in visual recovery by fenestration or shrinking of the scotoma, or both (8-10, 25).

9.3. Therapeutic window and current treatments

Most causative LHON mutations impair subunits of complex I of the mitochondrial respiratory chain and the therapeutic benefit of idebenone, which is a synthetic short-chain benzoquinone, is thought to be mediated by its ability to bypass the electron block at complex I, thus promoting ATP production (4). The effectiveness of this drug is mostly represented by the increased rate of recov-

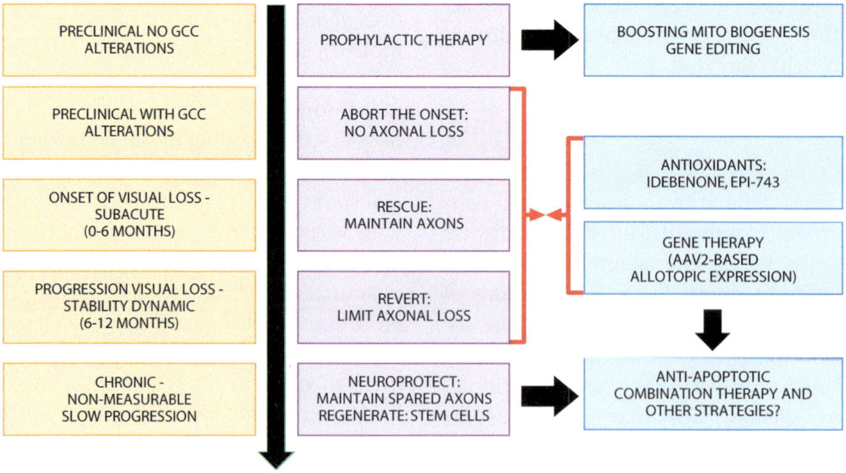

Figure 9.1: Therapeutic approaches to LHON depending on LHON disease stage.

ery in visual acuity after the "nadir", the so-called "*clinically relevant recovery*" (CRR), defined by visual acuity improvement from off-chart to on-chart, or on-chart recovery of at least two lines or 10 letters on the Early Treatment of Diabetic Retinopathy Study (ETDRS) chart (26). In a subgroup of treated patients, visual loss is somewhat stabilized, the so-called "*clinically relevant stabilization*" (CRS), which also leads to a better final visual outcome compared to the natural history (8-10, 26). When combined, CRR and CRS are referred to as "*clinically relevant benefit*" (CRB), and all these parameters have been used to define the effectiveness of idebenone in clinical studies (27).

Gene therapy is an obvious strategy to compensate for the defective mtDNA mutation and improve mitochondrial function. The attention has focused on the m.11778G>A mutation in *MT-ND4* given that it is the most common cause of LHON worldwide. All the published gene therapy trials indicate the same outcome, namely that it is not possible to abort the catastrophic loss of vision seen in the subacute stage and the improvement of vision is observed in the later stages. Similar to idebenone, once the nadir is reached, a substantial number of patients recover visual acuity, as defined by CRR and CRS, with the observed proportion experiencing visual recovery being significantly higher than what would be expected based on the natural history of historical treatment-naïve LHON cohorts (28). Two observations from the gene therapy trials are worth highlighting. Firstly, the trials were designed based on unilateral intravitreal injection of the gene therapy vector carrying the therapeutic *MT-ND4* transgene, under the assumption that the non-injected eye would serve as the control (29-31). The unexpected bilateral improvement resulted in the primary endpoint not being met, forcing the comparison with an external natural history cohort and all the associated possible sources of bias (28). Secondly, there is the somewhat counterintuitive observation that patients who were treated later, six months after disease onset, seemed to achieve a better final visual outcome compared with those who received the intravitreal injection of the gene therapy vector earlier, within six months of disease onset (29, 30, 32). The bilateral improvement has been proposed to arise due to the diffusion of the gene therapy vector from the injected eye to the contralateral non-injected eye, as partially supported by experiments on primates (29, 33). These are preliminary observations and further work is needed to substantiate this hypothesis.

Early-phase gene therapy studies for the m.3460G>A mtDNA LHON mutation is currently underway based on the similar principle of allotopic expression of a recoded version of the *MT-ND1* gene inserted into the nuclear genome, and the resulting mRNA having a mitochondrial targeting sequence (MTS) to direct the nascent protein to the mitochondrial compartment (https://clinicaltrials.gov/study/NCT05820152, accessed January 9 2024).

Conclusion

LHON is a paradigm for the field of mitochondrial medicine – the first disease to be defined on the molecular level and for which a therapy has been approved by the regulators. There are several unanswered mysteries, and resolving these will shed critical insight into the disease mechanisms driving RGC loss and optic nerve degeneration, and crucially, drive forward targeted therapeutic strategies backed by robust clinical trial design for this important cause of mitochondrial blindness.

References

1. Yu-Wai-Man P, Griffiths PG, Brown DT, Howell N, Turnbull DM, Chinnery PF. The epidemiology of Leber hereditary optic neuropathy in the North East of England. Am J Hum Genet. 2003 Feb;72(2):333-9.

2. Schaefer AM, McFarland R, Blakely EL, He L, Whittaker RG, Taylor RW, Chinnery PF, Turnbull DM. Prevalence of mitochondrial DNA disease in adults. Ann Neurol. 2008 Jan;63(1):35-9.

3. Wallace DC, Singh G, Lott MT, Hodge JA, Schurr TG, Lezza AM, Elsas LJ 2nd, Nikoskelainen EK. Mitochondrial DNA mutation associated with Leber's hereditary optic neuropathy. Science. 1988 Dec 9;242(4884):1427-30.

4. Amore G, Romagnoli M, Carbonelli M, Barboni P, Carelli V, La Morgia C. Therapeutic Options in Hereditary Optic Neuropathies. Drugs. 2021 Jan;81(1):57-86.

5. Newman NJ, Yu-Wai-Man P, Subramanian PS, Moster ML, Wang AG, Donahue SP, Leroy BP, Carelli V, Biousse V, Vignal-Clermont C, Sergott RC, Sadun AA, Rebolleda Fernández G, Chwalisz BK, Banik R, Bazin F, Roux M, Cox ED, Taiel M, Sahel JA; LHON REFLECT Study Group. Randomized trial of bilateral gene therapy

injection for m.11778G>A MT-ND4 Leber optic neuropathy. Brain. 2023 Apr 19;146(4):1328-1341.

6. Lam BL, Feuer WJ, Davis JL, Porciatti V, Yu H, Levy RB, Vanner E, Guy J. Leber Hereditary Optic Neuropathy Gene Therapy: Adverse Events and Visual Acuity Results of All Patient Groups. Am J Ophthalmol. 2022 Sep;241:262-271.

7. Yuan J, Zhang Y, Liu H, Wang D, Du Y, Tian Z, Li X, Yang S, Pei H, Wan X, Xiao S, Song L, Xiao X, Sun J, Wang Z, Li B. Seven-Year Follow-up of Gene Therapy for Leber's Hereditary Optic Neuropathy. Ophthalmology. 2020 Aug;127(8):1125-1127.

8. Carelli V, Ross-Cisneros FN, Sadun AA. Mitochondrial dysfunction as a cause of optic neuropathies. Prog Retin Eye Res. 2004 Jan;23(1):53-89.

9. Yu-Wai-Man P, Griffiths PG, Chinnery PF. Mitochondrial optic neuropathies - disease mechanisms and therapeutic strategies. Prog Retin Eye Res. 2011 Mar; 30(2):81-114.

10. Carelli V, Carbonelli M, de Coo IF, Kawasaki A, Klopstock T, Lagrèze WA, La Morgia C, Newman NJ, Orssaud C, Pott JWR, Sadun AA, van Everdingen J, Vignal-Clermont C, Votruba M, Yu-Wai-Man P, Barboni P. International Consensus Statement on the Clinical and Therapeutic Management of Leber Hereditary Optic Neuropathy. J Neuroophthalmol. 2017 Dec; 37(4):371-381. do

11. Barboni P, Carbonelli M, Savini G, Ramos Cdo V, Carta A, Berezovsky A, Salomao SR, Carelli V, Sadun AA. Natural history of Leber's hereditary optic neuropathy: longitudinal analysis of the retinal nerve fiber layer by optical coherence tomography. Ophthalmology. 2010 Mar;117(3):623-7.

12. Hwang TJ, Karanjia R, Moraes-Filho MN, Gale J, Tran JS, Chu ER, Salomao SR, Berezovsky A, Belfort R Jr, Moraes MN, Sadun F, DeNegri AM, La Morgia C, Barboni P, Ramos CDVF, Chicani CF, Quiros PA, Carelli V, Sadun AA. Natural History of Conversion of Leber's Hereditary Optic Neuropathy: A Prospective Case Series. Ophthalmology. 2017 Jun;124(6):843-850.

13. Lam BL, Feuer WJ, Schiffman JC, Porciatti V, Vandenbroucke R, Rosa PR, Gregori G, Guy J. Trial end points and natural history in patients with G11778A Leber hereditary optic neuropathy: preparation for gene therapy clinical trial. JAMA Ophthalmol. 2014 Apr 1; 132(4):428-36.

14. Nikoskelainen E, Hoyt WF, Nummelin K. Ophthalmoscopic findings in Leber's hereditary optic neuropathy. I. Fundus findings in asymptomatic family members. Arch Ophthalmol. 1982 Oct;100(10):1597-602.

15. Savini G, Barboni P, Valentino ML, Montagna P, Cortelli P, De Negri AM, Sadun F, Bianchi S, Longanesi L, Zanini M, Carelli V. Retinal nerve fiber layer evaluation by optical coherence tomography in unaffected carriers with Leber's hereditary optic neuropathy mutations. Ophthalmology. 2005 Jan;112(1):127-31.

16. Barboni P, Savini G, Feuer WJ, Budenz DL, Carbonelli M, Chicani F, Ramos Cdo V, Salomao SR, Negri AD, Parisi V, Carelli V, Sadun AA. Retinal nerve fiber layer thickness variability in Leber hereditary optic neuropathy carriers. Eur J Ophthalmol. 2012 Nov-Dec;22(6):985-91.

17. Carbonelli M, La Morgia C, Romagnoli M, Amore G, D'Agati P, Valentino ML, Caporali L, Cascavilla ML, Battista M, Borrelli E, Di Renzo A, Parisi V, Balducci N, Carelli V, Barboni P. Capturing the Pattern of Transition From Carrier to Affected in Leber Hereditary Optic Neuropathy. Am J Ophthalmol. 2022 Sep;241:71-79.

18. Balducci N, Savini G, Cascavilla ML, La Morgia C, Triolo G, Giglio R, Carbonelli M, Parisi V, Sadun AA, Bandello F, Carelli V, Barboni P. Macular nerve fibre and ganglion cell layer changes in acute Leber's hereditary optic neuropathy. Br J Ophthalmol. 2016 Sep;100(9): 1232-7.

19. Barboni P, Savini G, Valentino ML, Montagna P, Cortelli P, De Negri AM, Sadun F, Bianchi S, Longanesi L, Zanini M, de Vivo A, Carelli V. Retinal nerve fiber layer evaluation by optical coherence tomography in Leber's hereditary optic neuropathy. Ophthalmology. 2005 Jan;112(1):120-6.

20. Silva-Pinheiro P, Minczuk M. The potential of mitochondrial genome engineering. Nat Rev Genet. 2022 Apr;23(4):199-214.

21. Kim JS, Chen J. Base editing of organellar DNA with programmable deaminases. Nat Rev Mol Cell Biol. 2023 Oct 4.

22. Maresca A, Carelli V. Molecular Mechanisms behind Inherited Neurodegeneration of the Optic Nerve. Biomolecules. 2021 Mar 25;11(4):496.

23. Danese A, Patergnani S, Maresca A, Peron C, Raimondi A, Caporali L, Marchi S, La Morgia C, Del Dotto V, Zanna C, Iannielli A, Segnali A, Di Meo I, Cavaliere A, Lebiedzinska-Arciszewska M, Wieckowski MR, Martinuzzi A, Moraes-Filho MN, Salomao SR, Berezovsky A, Belfort R Jr, Buser C, Ross-Cisneros FN, Sadun AA, Tacchetti C, Broccoli V, Giorgi C, Tiranti V, Carelli V, Pinton P. Pathological mitophagy disrupts mitochondrial homeostasis in Leber's hereditary optic neuropathy. Cell Rep. 2022 Jul 19;40(3):111124.

24. Carelli V, La Morgia C, Ross-Cisneros FN, Sadun AA. Optic neuropathies: the tip of the neurodegeneration iceberg. Hum Mol Genet. 2017 Oct 1;26(R2):R139-R150.

25. Nakamura M, Yamamoto M. Variable pattern of visual recovery of Leber's hereditary optic neuropathy. Br J Ophthalmol. 2000 May;84(5):534-5.

26. Catarino CB, von Livonius B, Priglinger C, Banik R, Matloob S, Tamhankar MA, Castillo L, Friedburg C, Halfpenny CA, Lincoln JA, Traber GL, Acaroglu G, Black GCM, Doncel C, Fraser CL, Jakubaszko J, Landau K, Langenegger SJ, Muñoz-Negrete FJ, Newman NJ, Poulton J, Scoppettuolo E, Subramanian P, Toosy AT, Vidal M, Vincent AL, Votruba M, Zarowski M, Zermansky A, Lob F, Rudolph G, Mikazans O, Silva M, Llòria X, Metz G, Klopstock T. Real-World Clinical Experience With Idebenone in the Treatment of Leber Hereditary Optic Neuropathy. J Neuroophthalmol. 2020 Dec;40(4):558-565.

27. Yu-Wai-Man P, Carelli V, Newman NJ, Silva MJ, Linden A, Van Stavern G, Szaflik JP, Banik R, Lubinski W, Pemp B, Liao YJ, Subramanian PS, Misiuk-Hojlo M, Newman S, Castillo L, Kociecki J, Levin MH, Munoz-Negrete FJ, Yagan A, Cherninkova S, Katz D, Meunier A, Votruba M, Korwin M, Dziedziak J, Jurkute N, Harvey JP, La Morgia C, Priglinger C, Lloria X, Tomasso L, Klopstock T, LEROS Study Group. Therapeutic benefit of idebenone in patients with Leber hereditary optic neuropathy - The LEROS non-randomized controlled trial. Cell Rep Med. 2024;5(3):101437.

28. Carelli V, Newman NJ, Yu-Wai-Man P, Biousse V, Moster ML, Subramanian PS, Vignal-Clermont C, Wang AG, Donahue SP, Leroy BP, Sergott RC, Klopstock T, Sadun AA, Rebolleda Fernández G, Chwalisz BK, Banik R, Girmens JF, La Morgia C, DeBusk AA, Jurkute N, Priglinger C, Karanjia R, Josse C, Salzmann J, Montestruc F, Roux M, Taiel M, Sahel JA; the LHON Study Group. Indirect Comparison of Lenadogene Nolparvovec Gene Therapy Versus Natural History in Patients with Leber Hereditary Optic Neuropathy Carrying the m.11778G>A MT-ND4 Mutation. Ophthalmol Ther. 2023 Feb;12(1):401-429.

29. Yu-Wai-Man P, Newman NJ, Carelli V, Moster ML, Biousse V, Sadun AA, Klopstock T, Vignal-Clermont C, Sergott RC, Rudolph G, La Morgia C, Karanjia R, Taiel M, Blouin L, Burguière P, Smits G, Chevalier C, Masonson H, Salermo Y, Katz B, Picaud S, Calkins DJ, Sahel JA. Bilateral visual improvement with unilateral gene therapy injection for Leber hereditary optic neuropathy. Sci Transl Med. 2020 Dec 9;12(573):eaaz7423.

30. Newman NJ, Yu-Wai-Man P, Carelli V, Moster ML, Biousse V, Vignal-Clermont C, Sergott RC, Klopstock T, Sadun AA, Barboni P, DeBusk AA, Girmens JF, Rudolph G, Karanjia R, Taiel M, Blouin L, Smits G, Katz B, Sahel JA; LHON Study Group. Efficacy and Safety of Intravitreal Gene Therapy for Leber Hereditary Optic Neuropathy Treated within 6 Months of Disease Onset. Ophthalmology. 2021 May;128(5):649-660.

31. Lam BL, Feuer WJ, Davis JL, Porciatti V, Yu H, Levy RB, Vanner E, Guy J. Leber Hereditary Optic Neuropathy Gene Therapy: Adverse Events and Visual Acuity Results of All Patient Groups. Am J Ophthalmol. 2022 Sep;241:262-271.

32. Newman NJ, Yu-Wai-Man P, Subramanian PS, Moster ML, Wang AG, Donahue SP, Leroy BP, Carelli V, Biousse V, Vignal-Clermont C, Sergott RC, Sadun AA, Rebolleda Fernández G, Chwalisz BK, Banik R, Bazin F, Roux M, Cox ED, Taiel M, Sahel JA; LHON REFLECT Study Group. Randomized trial of bilateral gene therapy injection for m.11778G>A MT-ND4 Leber optic neuropathy. Brain. 2023 Apr 19;146(4):1328-1341.

33. Calkins DJ, Yu-Wai-Man P, Newman NJ, Taiel M, Singh P, Chalmey C, Rogue A, Carelli V, Ancian P, Sahel JA. Biodistribution of intravitreal lenadogene nolparvovec gene therapy in nonhuman primates. Mol Ther Methods Clin Dev. 2021 Oct1;23:307-318.

10. Idebenone treatment in LHON

Thomas Klopstock, Berthold Pemp, Valerio Carelli

10.1. What is idebenone?

Quinones are a family of natural and synthetic compounds that can, under certain circumstances, exhibit marked redox and antioxidant properties (1). Coenzyme Q10 (CoQ) is an endogenous quinone involved in several cellular processes, most importantly acting as an electron carrier in the mitochondrial respiratory chain and as an intramitochondrial antioxidant. The use of CoQ as an exogenous therapeutic is, however, hampered by its long lipophilic tail leading to low bioavailability and its relative inability to cross biological membranes.

Idebenone is a synthetic CoQ analogue (☞ Figure 10.1) with a much shorter and less lipophilic tail that allows efficient oral absorption and high permeability through biological membranes including those of cells and mitochondria. After reduction by NAD(P)H-quinone oxidoreductase 1 (NQO1) to its hydroquinone, it can capture electrons and transfer them directly to complex III of the respiratory chain, thus bypassing complex I, and also exerting antioxidant activity.

Idebenone was initially developed in Japan for the treatment of cognitive impairment in Alzheimer`s and cerebrovascular disease but a 1986 approval was withdrawn in 1998 due to lack of efficacy (2). Subsequently, the drug was investigated for several other disorders including Friedreich ataxia and Duchenne muscular dystrophy. The most convincing effects have, however, been found in LHON, and accordingly idebenone was approved by EMA for this indication in 2015.

10.2. Why idebenone is predestined to work in LHON

LHON is a paradigmatic complex I deficiency disorder. As outlined in Chapters 2., 4. and 8., almost all molecular causes of LHON compromise complex I of the respiratory chain, which in turn leads to increased oxidative stress and impaired electron flow to complex III, consequently reducing ATP production. Idebenone is exactly counteracting these pathomechanisms: it can shuttle electrons directly to complex III, thus bypassing the defective complex I and restoring downstream electron transfer and ultimately respiration, and it is a powerful intramitochondrial anti-oxidant.

10.3. Preclinical studies

In cybrids bearing the LHON-causing m.3460G>A mutation in the ND1 gene of the mtDNA and in carcinoma-derived cells bearing a truncating mutation in the same gene, idebenone, if maintained in the reduced state, could feed electrons to complex III (3). LHON fibroblast cell lines harbouring the m.11778G>A mutation in the ND4 gene of the mtDNA showed decreased cell growth, impaired ATP synthesis and elevated production of reactive oxygen species (ROS). The addition of idebenone could partially compensate these deleterious effects by increasing ATP production and reducing ROS levels (4). Besides its electron transfer and anti-oxidant capacities, idebenone has also shown to lower mitophagy rate in LHON cell models and to increase mitochondrial biogenesis available for compensatory energy production, both counteracting propensity to apoptosis (5, 6).

In a rodent cell culture of retinal ganglion cells (RGC), the tissue almost exclusively affected in LHON, exposure to the complex I inhibitor

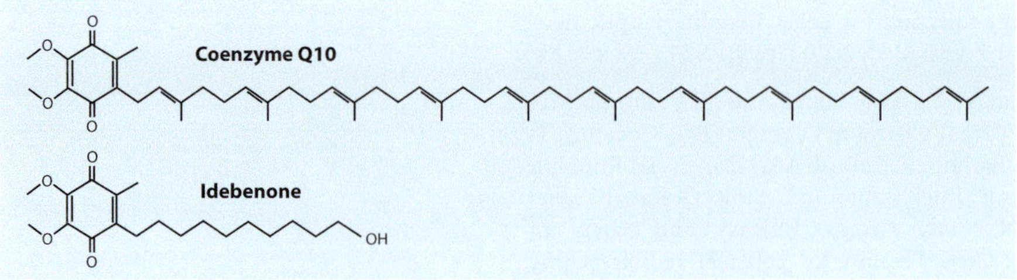

Figure 10.1: Idebenone chemical structure in comparison with CoQ.

rotenone leads to cell death that can be significantly rescued by preincubation with idebenone (7). In a toxic mouse model of LHON, generated by intravitreal injection of rotenone, orally administered idebenone penetrated well into the eye and protected against RGC death and retinal damage (7).

10.4. Clinical studies

These preclinical findings established the rationale to study idebenone in LHON patients. Subsequently to some suggestive case reports, a prospective, randomized, placebo-controlled parallel-group trial was conducted and published in 2011 (8), the "Rescue of Hereditary Optic Disease Outpatient Study" (RHODOS, NCT00747487). In short, 85 LHON patients harbouring one of the three common mutations and being within 5 years after onset of visual failure were randomized (2:1) to receive either idebenone 900mg/day or placebo for 24 weeks. While the primary endpoint, best recovery in visual acuity (i.e., the eye with the most beneficial delta between baseline and 24 weeks), did not reach statistical significance, there was a consistent trend in favor of idebenone as compared to placebo in all secondary endpoints (8). An observational follow-up study (RHODOS-OFU, NCT01421381) showed that the treatment effect persisted despite discontinuation of therapy for a median time of 30 months (9).

These findings were corroborated by a retrospective study comparing outcome in 44 idebenone-treated vs 59 untreated LHON patients (10). Clinically relevant recovery (CRR), defined as improvement of two lines of best corrected visual acuity (BCVA) on Early Treatment Diabetic Retinopathy Study (ETDRS) charts (or from off-chart to on-chart), occurred more often in the treated group (46 %) than in untreated patients (32 %). Similarly, a post-hoc analysis of the RHODOS trial showed a significantly higher CRR rate in patients under idebenone (30 %) vs. placebo (7 %).

Subsequently to the RHODOS trial, an international Expanded Access Program (EAP, NCT04381091) was set up to enable idebenone treatment of LHON patients within local regulations. This open-label analysis provided real world data for 111 LHON patients who started treatment within 1 year after onset of visual decline in the more recent eye. While treatment duration had been predefined as 6 months in the RHODOS trial, the EAP left it to the discretion of the treating physician which resulted in a mean treatment duration of 25.6 months. CRR in comparison to the nadir of vision was found in 46 % of 87 patients where longitudinal efficacy data were available (11). Time to initial observation of CRR varied between 2.5 and 26.5 months, with a mean of 9.5 months. The proportion of patients with CRR and the magnitude of recovery increased with treatment duration: more than half (55 %) of the patients with a CRR experienced their recovery after more than 6 months, and 90 % within 24 months of treatment. Average gain in BCVA for responders was 0.72 logarithm of the minimal angle of resolution (logMAR), equivalent to more than seven lines on the ETDRS chart. In addition to CRR, there was clinically relevant stabilization (CRS): 12 of 24 patients (50 %) maintained a visual acuity better than 1.0 logMAR from baseline to last visit (11).

The collated results of these studies eventually led in 2015 to the conditional approval (under exceptional circumstances) of idebenone (Raxone®) for the treatment of adolescent and adult LHON patients in the European Union.

Post-approval measures assigned by the European Medicine Agency (EMA) included a phase IV open-label intervention study with comparison to untreated patients from an external natural history control group (LEROS, NCT02774005) which was conducted at 31 study sites across nine European countries and the United States. In total, 199 LHON patients up to 5 years after symptom onset were treated with idebenone 900 mg/day. Outcomes were compared to an external natural history cohort of 372 patients, matched by time since symptom onset. The study confirmed the long-term efficacy of idebenone in the subacute/dynamic and chronic phases; however, the treatment effect varied depending on disease phase and the causative mtDNA mutation. The primary endpoint, predefined as clinically relevant benefit (CRB, a collation of CRR and CRS) after 12 months of treatment in the subacute/dynamic group, was met with 42.3 % [60/142] of treated eyes vs 20.7 % [40/193] of natural history eyes [p=0.002] (12).

10.5. Safety and efficacy of idebenone in LHON patients

Idebenone has shown a favorable safety profile in clinical studies: adverse events most frequently reported during treatment are gastrointestinal including mild diarrhea, transient headache, nasopharyngitis, cough and back pain. All severe adverse events in the EAP were classified as unrelated to treatment (11).

Regarding efficacy, roughly about half of the idebenone-treated LHON patients may be classified as non-responders. With the aim of exploring the possible reasons underlying unresponsiveness of these patients, a recent study revealed that two known polymorphic variants in the NQO1 gene, relatively frequent in the European population, drive idebenone efficacy *in vitro*. These variants are the rs1800566 (known by old nomenclature as c.609C>T), which defines the NQO1*2 allele (18.9 % of the European population), and the rs1131341 (known by old nomenclature as c.465C>T) defining the NQO1*3 allele (3.7 % of the European population). When these two variants are found homozygous, or in compound heterozygous combination, they consistently lower the cellular amount of NQO1 protein, ultimately hampering the complete reduction of idebenone administered to the cells (13). Under this condition, residual oxidized idebenone may variably cause ROS production and exert an inhibitory effect on mitochondrial respiration and cell viability (14). These observations open the possibility to better profiling the subpopulation of LHON patients who may benefit the most of idebenone therapy.

10.6. Treatment effects in chronic LHON

Many patients who start their treatment with idebenone in the early disease phase of subacute visual worsening experience a further decline of BCVA. This indicates that idebenone has limited capacity to stop the propagation of neuronal dysfunction in retinal ganglion cells and the optic nerve in subacute LHON. However, as seen in the studies summarized above, a recovery of vision after the so-called nadir occurs more often in treated than in untreated patients, supporting the ultimate neuroprotective properties of idebenone in LHON. A CRR is frequently achieved during the second year of the disease, when the patient has already reached the chronic stage of LHON, and sometimes even later on.

Subgroup analyses from the clinical trials RHODOS and LEROS, which included patients up to 5 years from disease onset, show that patients who started idebenone treatment in the chronic phase (i.e., 1-5 years after disease onset) also experience a CRR significantly more often than untreated patients. Effects of idebenone treatment when initiated later than 5 years after disease onset were investigated in some smaller studies (15, 16). A significant improvement in BCVA and visual field parameters was observed also in the late stage patients, but further investigations are necessary to validate these results.

Visual recovery in manifest optic atrophy requires that a part of the retinal ganglion cells and nerve fibers damaged during the active phase of LHON is not lost through apoptosis but only dysfunctional, allowing those cells to restore signal transduction later on. Besides its known actions in mitochondrial metabolism, idebenone could also play a role in promoting re-myelination of poorly myelinated viable axons in the optic nerve, which are detectable in tissue samples from LHON patients (17). In an animal model, orally administered idebenone has shown to increase the release of nerve growth factor in damaged brain tissue (18), which could stimulate this hypothetic treatment effect.

Taken together, these studies confirm that idebenone is safe and relatively effective in the treatment of LHON. An international consensus on timing and duration of the treatment was published in 2017 (19) but needs an update in light of the new study results.

References

1. Cores A, Carmona-Zafra N, Clerigue J, Villacampa M, Menendez JC. Quinones as Neuroprotective Agents. Antioxidants (Basel). 2023;12(7).

2. Meier T, Buyse G. Idebenone: an emerging therapy for Friedreich ataxia. Journal of neurology. 2009;256 Suppl 1:25-30.

3. Giorgio V, Petronilli V, Ghelli A, Carelli V, Rugolo M, Lenaz G, et al. The effects of idebenone on mitochondrial bioenergetics. Biochimica et biophysica acta. 2012; 1817(2):363-9.

4. Yu-Wai-Man P, Soiferman D, Moore DG, Burte F, Saada A. Evaluating the therapeutic potential of idebenone and related quinone analogues in Leber hereditary optic neuropathy. Mitochondrion. 2017;36:36-42.

5. Dombi E, Diot A, Morten K, Carver J, Lodge T, Fratter C, et al. The m.13051G>A mitochondrial DNA mutation results in variable neurology and activated mitophagy. Neurology. 2016;86(20):1921-3.

6. Danese A, Patergnani S, Maresca A, Peron C, Raimondi A, Caporali L, et al. Pathological mitophagy disrupts mitochondrial homeostasis in Leber's hereditary optic neuropathy. Cell Rep. 2022;40(3):111124.

7. Heitz FD, Erb M, Anklin C, Robay D, Pernet V, Gueven N. Idebenone protects against retinal damage and loss of vision in a mouse model of Leber's hereditary optic neuropathy. PLoS One. 2012;7(9):e45182.

8. Klopstock T, Yu-Wai-Man P, Dimitriadis K, Rouleau J, Heck S, Bailie M, et al. A randomized placebo-controlled trial of idebenone in Leber's hereditary optic neuropathy. Brain. 2011;134(Pt 9):2677-86.

9. Klopstock T, Metz G, Yu-Wai-Man P, Buchner B, Gallenmuller C, Bailie M, et al. Persistence of the treatment effect of idebenone in Leber's hereditary optic neuropathy. Brain. 2013;136(Pt 2):e230.

10. Carelli V, La Morgia C, Valentino ML, Rizzo G, Carbonelli M, De Negri AM, et al. Idebenone treatment in Leber's hereditary optic neuropathy. Brain. 2011; 134(Pt 9):e188.

11. Catarino CB, von Livonius B, Priglinger C, Banik R, Matloob S, Tamhankar MA, et al. Real-World Clinical Experience With Idebenone in the Treatment of Leber Hereditary Optic Neuropathy. Journal of neuro-ophthalmology : the official journal of the North American Neuro-Ophthalmology Society. 2020;40(4):558-65.

12. Yu-Wai-Man P, Carelli V, Newman NJ, Silva MJ, Linden A, Van Stavern G, et al. Therapeutic benefit of idebenone in patients with Leber hereditary optic neuropathy The LEROS non-randomized controlled trial. Cell Rep Med. 2024;5(3):101437.

13. Aleo SJ, Del Dotto V, Romagnoli M, Fiorini C, Capirossi G, Peron C, et al. Genetic variants affecting NQO1 protein levels impact the efficacy of idebenone treatment in Leber hereditary optic neuropathy. Cell Rep Med. 2024;101383.

14. Varricchio C, Beirne K, Heard C, Newland B, Rozanowska M, Brancale A, et al. The ying and yang of idebenone: Not too little, not too much - cell death in NQO1 deficient cells and the mouse retina. Free Radic Biol Med. 2020;152:551-60.

15. Pemp B, Kircher K, Reitner A. Visual function in chronic Leber's hereditary optic neuropathy during idebenone treatment initiated 5 to 50 years after onset. Graefes Arch Clin Exp Ophthalmol. 2019;257(12):2751-7.

16. Pemp B, Mitsch C, Kircher K, Reitner A. Changes in Visual Function and Correlations with Inner Retinal Structure in Acute and Chronic Leber's Hereditary Optic Neuropathy Patients after Treatment with Idebenone. J Clin Med. 2021;10(1).

17. Carelli V, Ross-Cisneros FN, Sadun AA. Mitochondrial dysfunction as a cause of optic neuropathies. Prog Retin Eye Res. 2004;23(1):53-89.

18. Nitta A, Murakami Y, Furukawa Y, Kawatsura W, Hayashi K, Yamada K, et al. Oral administration of idebenone induces nerve growth factor in the brain and improves learning and memory in basal forebrain-lesioned rats. Naunyn Schmiedebergs Arch Pharmacol. 1994;349(4):401-7.

19. Carelli V, Carbonelli M, de Coo IF, Kawasaki A, Klopstock T, Lagreze WA, et al. International Consensus Statement on the Clinical and Therapeutic Management of Leber Hereditary Optic Neuropathy. Journal of neuro-ophthalmology : the official journal of the North American Neuro-Ophthalmology Society. 2017;37(4): 371-81.

11. Gene therapy

Benson S. Chen, Thomas Klopstock, José-Alain Sahel, Patrick Yu-Wai-Man

Technological innovations within the field of gene therapy in the last 30 years have accelerated the development of treatments for a diverse range of inherited conditions (1). An increasing number of these treatments, including those for inherited retinal disorders, have been approved by regulators such as the European Medicines Agency, offering hope to patients affected by LHON. Gene therapy for the treatment of vision loss in LHON has been attractive to researchers since the identification of the first primary mutation causing LHON in 1988. LHON is an ideal disease for genetic intervention for several reasons (2). For most patients with LHON, a single gene defect responsible for the condition can be identified. In the eye, the gene defect typically affects only the RGCs, which can be accessed via the intravitreal (IVT) route. Finally, vision loss in LHON is acute and occurs sequentially, providing a natural time window for treatment to be initiated.

In this chapter we will review the development of gene therapy in LHON, beginning with a general overview of gene therapy. The scientific rationale for gene therapy in LHON and preclinical studies of allotopic expression will be discussed next, followed by the recent clinical trials aimed at the most common pathogenic mutation m.11778G>A in the *MT-ND4* gene. Finally, gene editing and future opportunities for gene therapy in LHON will be discussed.

11.1. Overview of gene therapy

Gene therapy refers to the technique of modifying an individual's genes to treat or cure disease. Broadly speaking, three mechanisms can be used:

- a disease-causing ("mutant") gene can be replaced with a healthy copy ("wild type") of the gene
- a disease-causing gene can be inactivated or "silenced" by introducing genetic material that interferes with its expression
- a new or modified gene can be introduced to help treat a disease.

Gene editing, which we discuss later, is a specific type of gene therapy that involves delivering genetic material that can edit pieces of DNA within a cell. Gene editing techniques can be used to introduce DNA corrections or integrate the correct DNA sequence that enables the gene to produce functional proteins; produce edits that activate a previously inactive silent gene; or silence or "knock-out" certain genes in a cell by altering or removing the problematic DNA sequence entirely.

A critical aspect of achieving therapeutic efficacy with gene therapy is maximising delivery of the genetic material into the target cells ("transduction"). Viral vectors are attractive, as viruses have a natural ability to deliver genetic material into cells. Five main classes of viral vectors have been tested for clinical applications: retroviruses, adenoviruses, adeno-associated viruses (AAV), lentiviruses, and herpes simplex virus. AAV is a preferred viral vector in ocular diseases because of its lack of pathogenicity, high transduction efficiency, and long-term expression of the transduced gene (the "transgene"). Over 100 different AAV serotypes have been described. Of the AAV serotypes that have been studied, AAV2/2, a hybrid AAV consisting of an AAV2 genome packaged into the capsid of another AAV2, has been shown to be highly efficient at transducing retinal ganglion cells (RGCs) via IVT injection (3-5).

11.2. Development of gene therapy in LHON – Allotopic expression

Most genetic mutations that cause LHON are point mutations in mitochondrial DNA (mtDNA), involving genes encoding subunits of respiratory complex I, the first enzyme of the respiratory chain located in the inner mitochondrial membrane. The defective subunit results in dysfunction of complex I and its many sequelae. From a theoretical basis, gene therapy for LHON would involve replacing the mutant gene by delivering the wild type gene into the mitochondria, which then undergoes transcription and translation into a functional protein to replace the defective complex I subunit. This process occurs in the mitochondrial matrix, involving the recruitment of different nuclear-encoded initiation, elongation, and termination factors.

The techniques used in the gene therapy of inherited autosomal disorders have limited application in mitochondrial disease. When conventional AAV vectors transduce a cell, the AAV vector particles are trafficked to the nucleus and not the mitochondria. Additionally, the mitochondrial double-membranes are relatively impervious and prevent the transfer of exogenous genetic material into the mitochondrial matrix. The outer mitochondrial membrane contains porins that only allow the passage of small molecules up to 5,000 Da in size; and translocase of the outer membrane (TOM), a complex of proteins that allow the movement of larger proteins that display a mitochondrial signal sequence. The TOM work in conjunction with translocase of the inner membrane (TIM), located in the inner mitochondrial membrane, to translocate proteins into the mitochondrion.

To overcome these challenges, earlier researchers developing gene therapy for LHON adopted the technique of allotopic expression as a treatment strategy (☞ Figure 11.1). First successfully demonstrated in yeast in the 1980s, allotopic expression involves the transcription and translation of a mitochondrial gene in the nuclear-cytosolic system (normally used by nuclear DNA) and importing the translated polypeptide into mitochondria with the assistance of a mitochondrial targeting sequence (MTS) recognized by the translocation membrane proteins. It is important to remember that the mitochondrial genetic code does not follow the rules of universal (nuclear) codon usage, with some codons specifying different amino acids in the mitochondrial code; so, the mitochondrial gene being allotopically expressed must be converted to the nuclear codon.

The first study demonstrating successful use of allotopic expression to rescue human cybrids containing the m.11778G>A mutation in *MT-ND4* was published in 2002 (6). Although the efficiency of allotopic expression was low, allotopically-rescued cybrids demonstrated increased complex I-dependent ATP synthesis compared to cybrids treated with a mock AAV. The success of these early *in vivo* experiments facilitated the development of animal models of LHON allowing the technique to be optimized further, alongside studies involving skin fibroblasts isolated from individuals affected by the m.11778G>A mutation (7). Important considerations included designing the nuclear-encoded *ND4* fusion gene with an MTS that would maximise import across the mitochondrial membrane and constructing a recombinant AAV (rAAV) with the best rate of RGC transduction. With further optimization, studies of allotopic expression of *ND4* in a rat model of LHON demonstrated prevention of RGC degeneration, preservation of complex I function in optic nerves, and preservation of visual function (8).

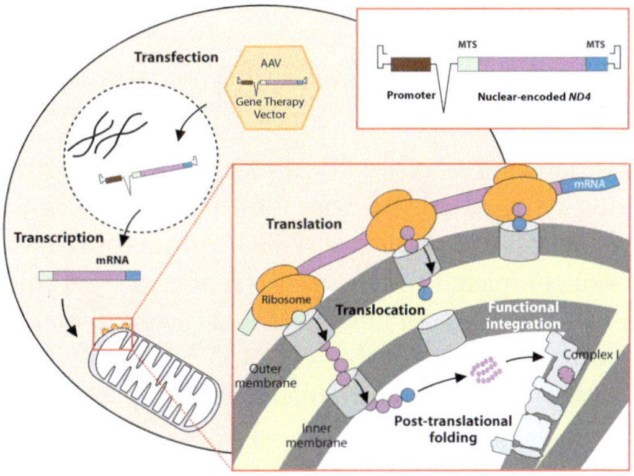

Figure 11.1: Gene therapy for LHON using the technique of allotopic expression. The gene therapy vector contains the replacement mitochondrial *ND4* gene modified according to the nuclear code. This nuclear-encoded version of *ND4* is fused to two mitochondrial targeting sequences (MTS) and a promoter is inserted for more efficient expression. The gene therapy vector is packaged into an adeno-associated virus (AAV), usually serotype 2, which is delivered to the retinal ganglion cells by intravitreal injection. The AAV transfects the retinal ganglion cells, delivering the gene therapy product into the nucleus. From here, the gene sequence undergoes transcription to messenger RNA (mRNA) and, with the aid of the MTS, directed to ribosomes on the external surface of the mitochondrial outer membrane, where gene translation occurs. As it is being synthesised, the newly translated ND4 polypeptide, aided by the MTS, is translocated through translocase of the outer and inner membrane (TOM and TIM, respectively) into the mitochondrial matrix. Finally, the imported ND4 subunit undergoes post-translational folding before being integrated within complex I, restoring its function.

11.3. Clinical trials of gene therapy in LHON

The success of the pre-clinical studies culminated in the first human trials of gene therapy for LHON in 2011, with open-label studies conducted by three separate groups involving participants carrying the m.11778G>A mutation in China, Europe, and the United States (4, 9-13). These studies confirmed the safety profile of allotopic *ND4* gene therapy. Although not specifically designed to demonstrate efficacy, these studies found that gene therapy appeared to be more efficacious for those treated within 12 months onset of visual loss, and sustained response in long-term follow-up. Unexpectedly, untreated eyes also demonstrated improved visual acuity.

To date, three Phase III clinical trials (and one long-term extension trial) for individuals with vision loss due to the m.11778G>A mutation have been completed and the results reported (☞ Table 11.1) (14-17). In all three trials, participants received IVT injection of rAAV2/2-*ND4* (also known as GS010 and lenadogene nolparvovec), with change in logMAR visual acuity the primary outcome measure.

The first Phase III clinical trial to be reported was 'REVERSE' (NCT02652780), a randomized, double-masked, sham-controlled, multicenter clinical trial, involving 37 participants with bilateral vision loss of 6-12 months duration (14). Each participant received an IVT injection of GS010 in one eye and sham treatment to the fellow eye. The second phase III clinical trial, 'RESCUE' (NCT02652767), was designed concurrently with the REVERSE trial, using similar assessment protocols and outcome measures; and included 38 participants with bilateral vision loss where the duration of vision loss for each eye was ≤6 months (17). A long-term follow-up study ('RESTORE') was conducted as an extension of REVERSE and RESCUE, with participants of both studies being followed for an additional three years, corresponding to five years post-treatment administration (16). The most recent phase III clinical trial of GS010, 'REFLECT' (NCT03293524), was a randomized, double-masked, placebo-controlled trial involving 98 patients with bilateral vision loss ≤1 year from onset, each receiving an intravitreal injection of GS010 in their first affected eye, and intravitreal injection of either GS010 or a placebo in their second affected eye (15).

The treatment effect of GS010 was consistent across all three studies, which also confirmed the earlier finding of improved visual acuity in untreated eyes. To probe the underlying mechanisms leading to bilateral improvement, a study was conducted using non-human primates (14). Three months after unilateral intravitreal injection of rAAV2/2-ND4, viral vector DNA was detected in all the tissue and fluid samples including the anterior segment, retina, and optic nerve of the contralateral untreated eye, as well as more posteriorly in the optic chiasm, optic tract, and lateral geniculate nucleus. The study's authors hypothesized that inter-eye transfer of the rAAV2/2-ND4 viral vector could be the result of transneuronal spread via the optic nerve and chiasm (14).

Although the REVERSE and RESCUE trials were designed for each participant to serve as their own control, the unexpected bilateral improvement in visual acuity meant that the magnitude of treatment effect could not be determined from trial results alone. Natural history studies have shown that a small proportion of patients experience some spontaneous improvement in visual acuity (18). To determine the magnitude of treatment effect of GS010, the visual acuity of 174 participants of the three clinical trials (and long-term extension trial) were pooled for further analysis compared to an external control group of 208 matched patients from 11 natural history studies (☞ Figure 11.2) (19). Compared to natural history patients, those who received treatment showed a mean improvement in visual acuity of –0.30 logMAR (equivalent to an improvement in 15 ETDRS letters) at last observation ($P<0.01$), with a maximal follow-up of 3.9 years after injection. Most treated eyes were on-chart (defined as a visual acuity better than 1.6 logMAR) compared to natural history eyes at 48 months after vision loss (89.6% versus 48.1%; $P<0.01$) and at last observation (76.1% versus 44.4%; $P<0.01$). After adjusting for age of onset, sex, ethnicity and follow-up duration, the estimated mean improvement in visual acuity was –0.43 logMAR (equivalent to an improvement of 21.5 ETDRS letters) compared to the natural-history-matched patients at last observation ($P<0.0001$) (19). Pooled analysis of 189 clinical trial participants receiving GS010 also confirmed

<table>
<tr><th>Study</th><th colspan="2">Main findings</th></tr>
<tr><td rowspan="4">REVERSE [NCT02652780](14)

37 participants, 6-12 months from onset of vision loss, received an intravitreal injection of GS010 in one eye and sham treatment in fellow eye</td><td colspan="2">Mean (±SD) visual acuity at baseline:</td></tr>
<tr><td>GS010-treated eyes:
1.67 (0.50) logMAR
(mean duration of vision loss: 8.8 months)</td><td>Sham-treated eyes:
1.55 (0.42) logMAR
(mean duration of vision loss: 9.3 months)</td></tr>
<tr><td colspan="2">Mean (±SD) change in visual acuity from baseline to week 96:</td></tr>
<tr><td>GS010-treated eyes:
–0.308 (0.068) logMAR
(+15 ETDRS letters)</td><td>Sham-treated eyes:
–0.259 (0.0608) logMAR
(+13 ETDRS letters)</td></tr>
<tr><td rowspan="6">RESCUE [NCT02652767] (17)

37 participants, within 6 months of onset of vision loss, received an intravitreal injection of GS010 in one eye and sham treatment in fellow eye</td><td colspan="2">Mean (±SD) visual acuity at baseline:</td></tr>
<tr><td>Sham-treated eyes:
1.31 (0.52) logMAR
(mean duration of vision loss: 108.5 days)</td><td>Sham-treated eyes:
1.26 (0.62) logMAR
(mean duration of vision loss: 115.8 days)</td></tr>
<tr><td colspan="2">Mean (±SD) change in visual acuity from baseline to week 96:</td></tr>
<tr><td>GS010-treated eyes:
+0.18 (0.12) logMAR
(–9 ETDRS letters)</td><td>Sham-treated eyes:
+0.21 (0.12) logMAR
(–10 ETDRS letters)</td></tr>
<tr><td colspan="2">Mean (±SD) change in visual acuity from nadir to week 96:</td></tr>
<tr><td>GS010-treated eyes:
–0.53 (0.08) logMAR
(+26 ETDRS letters)</td><td>Sham-treated eyes:
–0.46 (0.08) logMAR
(+23 ETDRS letters)</td></tr>
<tr><td rowspan="2">RESTORE [NCT03406104] (16)

Long-term follow-up of participants from REVERSE and RESCUE – see REVERSE and RESCUE above for baseline visual acuity data</td><td colspan="2">Mean (±SD) visual acuity from onset of vision loss:</td></tr>
<tr><td colspan="2">12 months (150 eyes): 1.57 (0.55) logMAR
18 months (149 eyes): 1.46 (0.51) logMAR
24 months (146 eyes): 1.40 (0.59) logMAR
36 months (128 eyes): 1.33 (0.59) logMAR
48 months (62 eyes): 1.26 (0.45) logMAR</td></tr>
<tr><td rowspan="10">REFLECT [NCT03293524] (15)

98 participants, within 12 months of onset of vision loss, received intravitreal injection of GS010 in first affected eye; second affected eye randomised to intravitreal injection of either GS010 or placebo</td><td colspan="2">Unilateral Treatment (50 participants)</td></tr>
<tr><td colspan="2">Mean change in visual acuity from baseline to 1.5 years:</td></tr>
<tr><td>GS010-treated eyes:
–0.21 (0.061) logMAR
(+11 ETDRS letters)</td><td>Placebo-treated eyes:
–0.04 (0.071) logMAR
(+2 ETDRS letters)</td></tr>
<tr><td colspan="2">Mean change in visual acuity from nadir to 1.5 years:</td></tr>
<tr><td>GS010-treated eyes:
–0.36 (0.049) logMAR
(+18 ETDRS letters)</td><td>Placebo-treated eyes:
–0.25 (0.041) logMAR
(+13 ETDRS letters)</td></tr>
<tr><td colspan="2">Bilateral Treatment (48 participants)</td></tr>
<tr><td colspan="2">Mean change in visual acuity from baseline to 1.5 years:</td></tr>
<tr><td>First GS010-treated eye:
–0.26 (0.063) logMAR
(+13 ETDRS letters)</td><td>Second GS010-treated eye:
–0.09 (0.072) logMAR
(+5 ETDRS letters)</td></tr>
<tr><td colspan="2">Mean change in visual acuity from nadir to 1.5 years:</td></tr>
<tr><td>First GS010-treated eye:
–0.38 (0.050) logMAR
(+19 ETDRS letters)</td><td>Second GS010-treated eye:
–0.31 (0.042) logMAR
(+16 ETDRS letters)</td></tr>
</table>

Table 11.1: Main finding of Phase III clinical trials for GS010.
ETDRS: Early Treatment Diabetic Retinopathy Study; logMAR: Logarithm of the Minimum Angle of Resolution; SD: standard deviation.

the long-term safety profile of the gene therapy product, with intraocular inflammation reported in 75.6% of GS010-treated eyes. Intraocular inflammation occurred in the anterior chamber or in the vitreous, was generally mild, and resolved with topical corticosteroids (20). Bio-dissemination of GS010 and systemic immune responses were limited.

The efficacy and safety of GS010 was also confirmed in a real-world setting, with 63 patients receiving GS010 through an early access program experiencing a mean improvement in visual acuity of −0.45logMAR (equivalent to an improvement of 22.5 ETDRS letters) in treated eyes at Year 1 (21). Intraocular inflammation occurred in 54 (42.9%) of treated eyes and was mild, lasting a mean of 155.8 days (21).

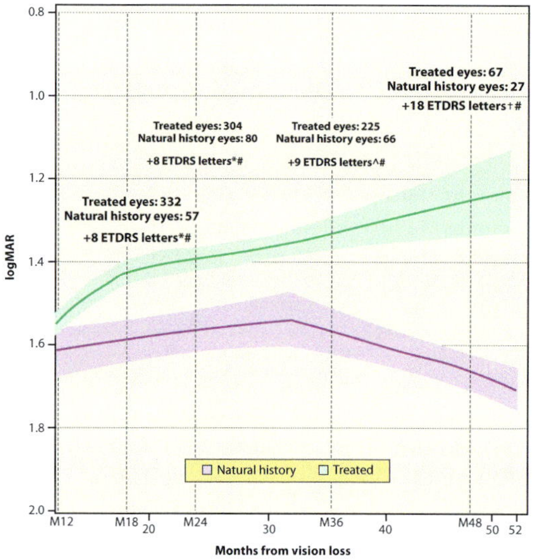

Figure 11.2: The evolution of visual acuities from 12 months after onset of vision loss for GS010-treated eyes (n=348) and natural history eyes (n=408) estimated by locally estimated scatterplot smoothing (LOESS) regression (solid line) with 95% confidence interval around the fitted curve (shaded area). Mean differences in visual acuity at months 18, 24, 36, and 48 were estimated by a mixed-model analysis of covariance (ANCOVA) demonstrating a significant difference in favor of GS010-treated eyes (**P*=0.03; ^*P*=0.02; †*P*<0.01; and # Kruskal Wallis test, *P*<0.01). Adapted from Carelli et al. *Ophthalmol Ther* 2023;12(1):401-29.

11.4. Gene therapy – Looking to the future

At this time, GS010 (trade name LUMEVOQ®) remains an experimental therapy that has not yet received market authorisation for use in Europe or the United States. Even if approved, only individuals carrying the m.11778G>A mutation would be eligible for treatment. For those carrying a different mutation, there remains significant unmet needs. Individuals with chronic LHON (vision loss >12 months duration), who represent the vast majority of those affected by LHON, also have significant unmet needs. The efficacy of gene therapy for chronic LHON has only been investigated in early phase studies with mixed results. An upcoming Phase II/III clinical trial in the United Kingdom will investigate the effect of GS010 in patients carrying the m.11778G>A mutation with chronic LHON, with vision loss duration between >12 months and <5 years.

Research attention has shifted to therapies for individuals carrying other LHON-causing mutations, in particular m.3460G>A in *MT-ND1* and m.11484T>C in *MT-ND6*. There is interest in studying allotopic expression of *ND1* and *ND6*, but also using new strategies including delivery of the transgene to the mitochondria using a modified AAV, where one of the viral capsid proteins is modified to include an MTS ("MTS-AAV") (22). Similar to the MTS that directs the cytoplasmically synthesised protein to the mitochondria, the MTS directs the AAV to the mitochondria where the packaged gene can be delivered. The MTS-AAV approach may be more efficient than allotopic expression, as the wild type mtDNA gene does not require modification to the nuclear code, nor is a separate import and assembly pathway required.

Developments in gene therapies for other mitochondrial diseases also have potential application for the treatment of LHON. One area of interest, still in the pre-clinical phase, is the use of gene editing. Although gene editing with clustered regularly interspaced short palindromic repeats (CRISPR) systems has been discussed as a revolutionary tool for gene editing, current CRISPR systems that utilize a guide RNA are ineffective because mitochondria do not readily import RNA (23). Mitochondrially-targeted zinc finger nucleases (ZFNs) and transcription activator-like effector nucleases

(TALENs) have been used successfully *in vitro* and in animal models to induce heteroplasmic shift and reduce the load of mutant mtDNA in cells (23). However, this strategy has limited applicability for LHON as most carriers are homoplasmic mutant. One potential application is the utilization of ZFNs and TALENs to induce heteroplasmy shift in oocytes or embryos containing high levels of the pathogenic mtDNA variant prior to implantation, thereby preventing transmission of LHON to the next generation (24). Another genomic approach that is being considered is mitochondrial base editing using non-CRISPR-based mtDNA editing tools, including Ddda-derived cytosine base editor (DdCBE) (25, 26). The platform is still in its infancy and is currently limited to CG-to-TA editing, making it a viable strategy only for the m.14484T>C mutation in *MT-ND6*.

Pre-clinical research is also focused on using gene therapy to introduce new or modified genes to treat disease. This approach to gene therapy is being investigated in several neurodegenerative diseases, including glaucoma. Here, gene therapy is directed at introducing genes involved in the regulation of mitochondrial biogenesis and neuronal survival. Specific genes under pre-clinical investigation that have been shown to improve defective mitochondrial function and/or increase neuronal survival include *NDI1*, *NRF2*, *SIRT1*, *SOD2*, and a novel transgene coding brain derived neurotrophic factor (BDNF) and tropomyosin-related receptor-B (TrKB) (3, 27-31). In contrast to mutation-specific therapies that are focused on gene replacement or gene editing, these mutation-independent therapies are incredibly advantageous as, theoretically, most patients with LHON would be eligible for treatment.

Conclusion

Genetic therapies hold great promise for individuals affected by LHON. Advances in gene delivery systems and gene editing technology have facilitated the development of innovative therapies over the past decade, the most notable being allotopically expressed *ND4* for the treatment of LHON due to the m.11778G>A mutation. Given the rarity of LHON and the costs associated with the development of gene therapy products, increasing effort is being directed towards treatment strategies that are mutation independent. For these treatments to have translational success from bench to bedside, a collaborative approach is required, synchronising the efforts and actions of academia, funding agencies, the pharmaceutical and biotechnology industry, patient advocacy groups, and policy makers. With the number of therapies on the horizon for LHON access to rapid genetic testing is critical, in order to establish the molecular diagnosis, assess clinical trial eligibility, and access treatment.

References

1. Dunbar CE, High KA, Joung JK, Kohn DB, Ozawa K, Sadelain M. Gene therapy comes of age. Science 2018; 359:6372.

2. Chen BS, Yu-Wai-Man P, Newman NJ. Developments in the treatment of Leber hereditary optic neuropathy. Curr Neurol Neurosci Rep 2022;22(12):881-892.

3. Chadderton N, Palfi A, Millington-Ward S, et al. Intravitreal delivery of AAV-NDI1 provides functional benefit in a murine model of Leber hereditary optic neuropathy. Eur J Hum Genet 2013;21(1):62-8.

4. Vignal C, Uretsky S, Fitoussi S, et al. Safety of rAAV2/2-ND4 gene therapy for Leber hereditary optic neuropathy. Ophthalmology 2018;125(6):945-47.

5. Yin L, Greenberg K, Hunter JJ, et al. Intravitreal injection of AAV2 transduces macaque inner retina. Invest Ophthalmol Vis Sci 2011;52(5):2775-83.

6. Guy J, Qi X, Pallotti F, et al. Rescue of a mitochondrial deficiency causing Leber hereditary optic neuropathy. Ann Neurol 2002;52(5):534-42.

7. Bonnet C, Augustin S, Ellouze S, et al. The optimized allotopic expression of ND1 or ND4 genes restores respiratory chain complex I activity in fibroblasts harboring mutations in these genes. Biochim Biophys Acta 2008; 1783(10):1707-17.

8. Cwerman-Thibault H, Augustin S, Lechauve C, et al. Nuclear expression of mitochondrial ND4 leads to the protein assembling in complex I and prevents optic atrophy and visual loss. Mol Ther Methods Clin Dev 2015;2: 15003.

9. Feuer WJ, Schiffman JC, Davis JL, et al. Gene therapy for Leber hereditary optic neuropathy: Initial results. Ophthalmology 2016;123(3):558-70.

10. Guy J, Feuer WJ, Davis JL, et al. Gene therapy for Leber hereditary optic neuropathy: Low- and medium-dose visual results. Ophthalmology 2017;124(11):1621-34.

11. Lam BL, Feuer WJ, Davis JL, et al. Leber hereditary optic neuropathy gene therapy: Adverse events and vi-

sual acuity results of all patient groups. Am J Ophthalmol 2022;241:262-271.

12. Vignal-Clermont C, Girmens JF, Audo I, et al. Safety of intravitreal gene therapy for treatment of subjects with Leber hereditary optic neuropathy due to mutations in the mitochondrial ND4 gene: The REVEAL Study. BioDrugs 2021;35(2):201-14.

13. Wan X, Pei H, Zhao MJ, et al. Efficacy and safety of rAAV2-ND4 treatment for Leber's hereditary optic neuropathy. Sci Rep 2016;6:21587.

14. Yu-Wai-Man P, Newman NJ, Carelli V, et al. Bilateral visual improvement with unilateral gene therapy injection for Leber hereditary optic neuropathy. Sci Transl Med 2020;12(573):eaaz7423.

15. Newman NJ, Yu-Wai-Man P, Subramanian PS, et al. Randomized trial of bilateral gene therapy injection for m.11778G > A MT-ND4 Leber optic neuropathy. Brain 2023;146(4):1328-1341.

16. Biousse V, Newman NJ, Yu-Wai-Man P, et al. Long-term follow-up after unilateral intravitreal gene therapy for Leber hereditary optic neuropathy: The RESTORE Study. J Neuroophthalmol 2021;41(3):309-15.

17. Newman NJ, Yu-Wai-Man P, Carelli V, et al. Efficacy and safety of intravitreal gene therapy for Leber hereditary optic neuropathy treated within 6 months of disease onset. Ophthalmology 2021;128(5):649-60.

18. Newman NJ, Carelli V, Taiel M, Yu-Wai-Man P. Visual outcomes in Leber hereditary optic neuropathy patients with the m.11778G>A (MTND4) mitochondrial DNA mutation. J Neuroophthalmol 2020;40(4):547-57.

19. Carelli V, Newman NJ, Yu-Wai-Man P, et al. Indirect comparison of lenadogene nolparvovec gene therapy versus natural history in patients with Leber hereditary optic neuropathy carrying the m.11778G>A MT-ND4 mutation. Ophthalmol Ther 2023;12(1):401-29.

20. Vignal-Clermont C, Yu-Wai-Man P, Newman NJ, et al. Safety of lenadogene nolparvovec gene therapy over 5 years in 189 patients with Leber hereditary optic neuropathy. Am J Ophthalmol 2023;249:108-125.

21. Vignal-Clermont C, Carelli V, Hage R, et al. Use of lenadogene nolparvovec gene therapy for Leber hereditary optic neuropathy in early access programs. North American Neuro-Ophthamology Society 49th Annual Meeting. Orlando, FL, USA, 2023.

22. Liu Y, Eastwood JD, Alba DE, et al. Gene therapy restores mitochondrial function and protects retinal ganglion cells in optic neuropathy induced by a mito-targeted mutant ND1 gene. Gene Ther 2022;29(6):368-378.

23. Jackson CB, Turnbull DM, Minczuk M, Gammage PA. Therapeutic manipulation of mtDNA heteroplasmy: A Shifting Perspective. Trends Mol Med 2020;26(7):698-709.

24. Reddy P, Ocampo A, Suzuki K, et al. Selective elimination of mitochondrial mutations in the germline by genome editing. Cell 2015;161(3):459-69.

25. Mok BY, de Moraes MH, Zeng J, et al. A bacterial cytidine deaminase toxin enables CRISPR-free mitochondrial base editing. Nature 2020;583(7817):631-37.

26. Mok BY, Kotrys AV, Raguram A, Huang TP, Mootha VK, Liu DR. CRISPR-free base editors with enhanced activity and expanded targeting scope in mitochondrial and nuclear DNA. Nat Biotechnol 2022;40(9):1378-1387.

27. Khatib TZ, Osborne A, Yang S, et al. Receptor-ligand supplementation via a self-cleaving 2A peptide-based gene therapy promotes CNS axonal transport with functional recovery. Sci Adv 2021;7(14).

28. Liang KJ, Woodard KT, Weaver MA, Gaylor JP, Weiss ER, Samulski RJ. AAV-Nrf2 promotes protection and recovery in animal models of oxidative stress. Mol Ther 2017;25(3):765-79.

29. Marella M, Seo BB, Thomas BB, Matsuno-Yagi A, Yagi T. Successful amelioration of mitochondrial optic neuropathy using the yeast NDI1 gene in a rat animal model. PLoS One 2010;5(7):e11472.

30. Qi X, Sun L, Hauswirth WW, Lewin AS, Guy J. Use of mitochondrial antioxidant defenses for rescue of cells with a Leber hereditary optic neuropathy-causing mutation. Arch Ophthalmol 2007;125(2):268-72.

31. Ross AG, Chaqour B, McDougald DS, et al. Selective upregulation of SIRT1 expression in retinal ganglion cells by AAV-mediated gene delivery increases neuronal cell survival and alleviates axon demyelination associated with optic neuritis. Biomolecules 2022;12(6).

Index

R

S

T

V